Free Video  **Free Video**

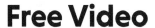

Essential Test Tips Video from Trivium Test Prep

Dear Customer,

Thank you for purchasing from Trivium Test Prep! We're honored to help you prepare for your PTCB exam.

To show our appreciation, we're offering a **FREE *PTCB Essential Test Tips* Video by Trivium Test Prep.*** Our video includes 35 test preparation strategies that will make you successful on the PTCB. All we ask is that you email us your feedback and describe your experience with our product. Amazing, awful, or just so-so: we want to hear what you have to say!

To receive your **FREE *PTCB Essential Test Tips* Video**, please email us at 5star@triviumtestprep.com. Include "Free 5 Star" in the subject line and the following information in your email:

1. The title of the product you purchased.
2. Your rating from 1 – 5 (with 5 being the best).
3. Your feedback about the product, including how our materials helped you meet your goals and ways in which we can improve our products.
4. Your full name and shipping address so we can send your **FREE *PTCB Essential Test Tips* Video**.

If you have any questions or concerns please feel free to contact us directly at 5star@triviumtestprep.com.

Thank you!

–Trivium Test Prep Team

*To get access to the free video please email us at 5star@triviumtestprep.com, and please follow the instructions above.

PTCB PRACTICE EXAM BOOK 2020 – 2021

4 Full-Length Practice Tests for the Pharmacy Technician Certification Board Examination

TABLE OF CONTENTS

INTRODUCTION: BECOMING A CERTIFIED PHARMACY TECHNICIAN

The PTCB's Pharmacy Technician Certification Exam (PTCE) is accredited by the National Commission for Certifying Agencies (NCCA). To schedule a test, you must first get authorization from the PTCB showing you have met all the pre-qualifications. The pre-qualifications are explained in the PTCB Code of Conduct shown at the end of this chapter. After you receive authorization and pay the $129 test fee, you can schedule a test online or by phone with Pearson-VUE Professional Testing Centers. When you arrive at the center, be sure to have photo identification to prove your identity. The testing center may also collect your palm vein image digitally for verification and to protect the integrity of the test. No personal items are allowed in the testing area; you will be assigned a locker to secure your items while you test. When you enter the testing area, an employee will sign you in to a computer workstation and hand you any other materials permitted only for testing purposes. You are monitored at all times while taking the test and cannot communicate with other test-takers. Any disruptive or fraudulent behavior can cause termination of testing.

The PTCE is a computer-generated multiple-choice exam that contains ninety questions. Of the ninety questions, eighty questions are scored and ten questions are unscored. There are four possible answers for each question, but only one is correct. The exam takes 2 hours. A score of 1400/1600 or better is required to pass the exam. The range of possible scores is between 1000 and 1600 and is based off of the Modified Angoff method of testing. You will officially know if you passed the test within 1 to 3 weeks after you take the exam. Within 6 weeks, you will be sent an official certificate and wallet card stating you are a certified pharmacy technician.

WHAT IS THE PTCB?

The main governing organization for the Pharmacy Technician Certification Exam (PTCE) is the **Pharmacy Technician Certification Board (PTCB)**. The

PTCB was created in 1995 by leaders in both the American Society of Health Systems Pharmacists (ASHP) and the American Pharmacist Association (APA). These leaders, realizing the need for a better way to educate pharmacy technicians on the skill sets essential to their profession, created a board of advisors who initiated a testing system that assesses the knowledge and abilities needed to perform pharmacy technician work responsibilities.

By passing the PTCE, pharmacy technicians are nationally accredited and receive the title of a Certified Pharmacy Technician, or CPhT. This accreditation proves to employers that its holder's knowledge will be beneficial to their company. The skill sets tested on the exam specifically correspond to required knowledge for performing technical and production duties in the pharmacy.

WHAT YOU NEED TO KNOW TO PASS THE PTCE

To pass the PTCE, the PTCB requires knowledge of specific subjects related to work as a pharmacy technician. The subjects and the percentage of each subject that will be on the test are listed below:

Pharmacology (13.75%): brand and generic names of pharmaceuticals, therapeutic equivalence, strength/dose, dosage forms, physical appearance, routes of administration, duration of drug therapy, drug interactions, common and severe/adverse side effects, allergies, therapeutic contraindications, dosage and indication of legend, OTC medications, herbal and dietary supplements

Pharmacy Law and Ethics (12.50%): storage, handling, and disposal of hazardous substances; hazardous substance exposure (including prevention and treatment); controlled substance transfer regulations; controlled substance documentation for receiving, ordering, returning, loss/theft, and destruction; formula to verify the validity of DEA numbers, record keeping, documentation, and record retention; restricted drug programs and related prescription processing requirements; professional standards related to HIPAA; requirements for consultation; recalls; infection control; professional standards; reconciliation between state and federal laws; facility, equipment, and supply requirements

Medication Safety (12.50%): error prevention strategies, patient package insert and medication guide requirements, look-alike/sound-alike medications, high-alert/high-risk medications, common safety strategies, issues that require pharmacist intervention

Sterile and Non-Sterile Compounding (8.75%): infection control, handling and disposal requirements, product stability, equipment and supplies, sterile compounding process, non-sterile compounding process

Quality Assurance (7.50%): quality assurance practices and inventory control, infection control documentation, risk management guidelines and regulations, production, efficacy and customer satisfaction measures

Medication Order Entry and Fill Process (17.50%): order entry; intake, interpretation, and data entry; calculate doses required; fill process; labeling requirements; packaging requirements; dispensing process

Inventory Management (8.75%): define NDC, lot numbers, expiration dates, formulary product list, ordering and receiving, storage and removal

Billing and Reimbursement (8.75%): reimbursement policy and plans, third-party resolution, third-party reimbursement, healthcare reimbursement, coordination of benefits

Information System Usage and Application (10.00%): pharmacy-related computer applications, databases, documentation management, inventory reports, override reports, diversion reports, patient adherence, risk factors, drug allergies, side effects, electronic medical records

Pharmacy Math and Calculations: dispersed throughout other subject areas including inventory, compounding, billing and reimbursement, order entry and fill process, and pharmacology

AFTER THE PTCE

After you pass the PTCE, you will receive your certification by mail. To keep your certification current, you will be required to re-certify every 2 years. Because CPhTs are expanding their roles to better support pharmacists, changes have taken place in 2015 and 2016. Since 2015, CPhTs have been required to submit pharmacy technician-specific continuing education (CE) hours. For reinstatement, pharmacy technicians must submit 20 CE hours. Of the 20 CE hours, 2 CE hours must be in pharmacy law, and 1 CE hour must be in patient safety. As of January 1, 2016, only 10 of the total 20 CE hours may be accredited by passing a college-based equivalent course with a grade of "C." Certificate holders must also pay a reinstatement fee every 2 years.

Depending on your state, you may also be required to re-register every 2 years. Registration is state specific, and it is important to check with your state board of pharmacy and/or department of health to determine the requirements for re-registration in your state. Most states require their own set of CE hours and a re-registration fee.

Due to the professional standards of working in a pharmacy, drug-related offenses and felonies as well as other disciplinary issues may cause suspension and revocation of your license and certification. Remember that you are a trusted professional and must abide by a set of ethical standards. When you become PTCB certified, you will take an oath to uphold the PTCB Code of Conduct.

The Code of Conduct follows:

PTCB is dedicated to providing and implementing appropriate standards designed to serve pharmacy technicians, employers, pharmacists, and patients. First and foremost, PTCB certificants and candidates give priority to the health interests and protection of the public, and act in a manner that promotes integrity and reflects positively on the work of pharmacy technicians, consistent with appropriate ethical and legal standards.

As pharmacy technicians, and under the supervision of a licensed pharmacist, PTCB certificants and candidates have the obligation to: maintain high standards of integrity and conduct; accept responsibility for their actions; continually seek to improve their performance in the workplace; practice with fairness and honesty; and, encourage others to act in an ethical manner consistent with the standards and responsibilities set forth below. Pharmacy technicians assist pharmacists in dispensing medications and remain accountable to supervising pharmacists with regard to all pharmacy activities, and will act consistent with all applicable laws and regulations.

A. Responsibilities Relating to Legal Requirements.

Each certificant/candidate must:

1. Act consistent with all legal requirements relating to pharmacy technician practice, including Federal, State, and local laws and regulations.

2. Refrain from any behavior that violates legal or ethical standards, including all criminal laws, Federal laws and agency regulations, and State laws and regulatory agency rules.

B. Responsibilities to PTCB/Compliance with Organizational Policies and Rules.

Each certificant/candidate must:

1. Act consistent with all applicable PTCB Policies and requirements.

2. Provide accurate, truthful, and complete information to PTCB.

3. Maintain the security and confidentiality of PTCB Examination information and materials, including the prevention of unauthorized disclosure of test items and format and other confidential information.

4. Cooperate with PTCB concerning conduct review matters, including the submission of all required information in a timely, truthful, and accurate manner.

5. Report to PTCB apparent violations of this Code upon a reasonable and clear factual basis.

C. Responsibilities to the Public and Employers.

Each certificant/candidate must:

1. Deliver competent, safe, and appropriate pharmacy and related services.

2. Recognize practice limitations and provide services only when qualified and authorized by a supervising pharmacist and consistent with applicable laws and regulations. The certificant/candidate is responsible for determining the limits of his/her own abilities based on legal requirements, training, knowledge, skills, experience, and other relevant considerations.

3. Maintain and respect the confidentiality of sensitive information obtained in the course of all work and pharmacy-related activities, as directed by the supervising pharmacist and consistent with legal requirements, unless: the information is reasonably understood to pertain to unlawful activity; a court or governmental agency lawfully directs the release of the information; the patient or the employer expressly authorizes the release of specific information; or, the failure to release such information would likely result in death or serious physical harm to employees and/or patients.

4. Use pharmacy technician credentials properly, and provide truthful and accurate representations concerning education, experience, competency, and the performance of services.

5. Provide truthful and accurate representations to the public and employers.

6. Follow appropriate health and safety procedures with respect to all pharmacy-related activities and duties.

7. Protect the public, employees, and employers from conditions where injury and damage are reasonably foreseeable.

8. Disclose to patients or employers significant circumstances that could be construed as a conflict of interest or an appearance of impropriety.

9. Avoid conduct that could cause a conflict of interest with the interests of a patient or employer.

10. Assure that a real or perceived conflict of interest does not compromise legitimate interests of a patient or employer, and does not influence or interfere with work-related judgments.

Code of Conduct, Pharmacy Technician Certification Board, 2014, https://www.ptcb.org/resources/code-of-conduct

ONE: Practice Test One

READ THE QUESTION CAREFULLY AND CHOOSE THE MOST CORRECT ANSWER.

1. Which of the following is the drug suffix used for histamine-2 blockers?

    A) –olol

    B) –pril

    C) –tidine

    D) –artan

2. What is the weight limit of a Class A balance?

    A) 240 mg

    B) 120 mg

    C) 100 mg

    D) 360 mg

3. Which of the following is NOT considered a possible abbreviation error based on the Joint Commission's Do Not Use list?

    A) using cc (cubic centimeter) instead of mL (milliliter)

    B) using apothecary units instead of metric units

    C) using STAT to mean as soon as possible

    D) using MS interchangeably to mean both morphine sulfate and magnesium sulfate

4. Barcode administration technology

    A) reduces medication errors on the patient's label by matching the inpatient's information on their wristband and verifying by scanning the information before medication is administered.

    B) tracks patient compliance in taking maintenance medications and tracks disease management through software systems connected to physicians' offices, hospitals, and pharmacies.

    C) is used to unit-dose medications in stock bottles in the centralized pharmacy.

    D) includes automatic pumping systems that can compound several sterile ingredients into a finished solution dispensed in a single patient bag without being manually touched by the technician.

5. The drug *ondansetron* is used for

    A) pain.

    B) diabetes.

    C) stomach acid.

    D) nausea.

6. Which is a disease or condition of the musculoskeletal system?

   A) leukemia

   B) cystitis

   C) angina

   D) osteoarthritis

7. Approximately how many medication errors occur in the United States each year?

   A) 3 million

   B) 5 million

   C) 1.5 million

   D) 2.5 million

8. The BIN number on a health insurance card

   A) is used by PBMs for network benefit routing and may change depending on what benefit is being billed.

   B) directs the claim to the correct third-party provider.

   C) directs the claim to the specific insurance benefits for that group.

   D) is used as an identification tool along with the dates of birth of each person covered, which are listed on the card.

9. How is 2014 written in roman numerals?

   A) MMCCVI

   B) MMXIV

   C) MMCXIV

   D) MMXVI

10. The root word *lapar/o* means

    A) liver.

    B) abdomen.

    C) body tissue.

    D) breast.

11. Which of the following is NOT required on a non-controlled hard copy?

    A) patient's name

    B) prescriber's DEA number

    C) patient's phone number

    D) prescriber's name

12. What does the drug *salmeterol* do?

    A) It prevents asthma attacks and bronchospasms.

    B) It is used to lower fevers and treat inflammation.

    C) It is used to treat autoimmune disorders.

    D) It is an estrogen modulator.

13. What chapter of the USP addresses non-sterile compounding?

    A) 795

    B) 799

    C) 797

    D) 796

14. What is the answer to $\frac{3}{8} + \frac{2}{5}$ in fractions?

    A) $\frac{31}{40}$

    B) $\frac{25}{40}$

    C) $\frac{12}{40}$

    D) $\frac{15}{40}$

15. Harvey Wiley, the chief chemist for the Bureau of Chemistry, helped to pass which act?

    A) the Pure Food and Drug Act of 1906

    B) the Food, Drug, and Cosmetic Act of 1938

    C) the Poison Prevention Packaging Act

    D) the Harrison Narcotics Tax Act of 1914

16. Which of the following is the definition of the suffix –stomy?
    A) incision
    B) formation
    C) abnormal condition
    D) artificial opening

17. Which is not considered a managed care plan?
    A) POS plan
    B) HMOs
    C) PPOs
    D) PAPs

18. Medication errors are the _____ leading cause of preventable death and injuries in the United States.
    A) first
    B) fifth
    C) fourth
    D) third

19. 3,600 mL is equivalent to how many L?
    A) 360 L
    B) 36 L
    C) 3.6 L
    D) 0.36 L

20. Pharmacodynamics
    A) is how the action, effect, and breakdown of drugs happens in the body.
    B) is the difference in quantity of medication between the effective dose and the amount that causes adverse side effects.
    C) is when two drugs have the same bioavailability.
    D) is not applicable if a patient decides not to take a drug the physician prescribes.

21. In which year was the Food and Drug Administration formed?
    A) 1906
    B) 1938
    C) 1862
    D) 1901

22. Which medication error occurs when the prescribed dose is not administered as ordered?
    A) wrong dosage form errors
    B) improper dose errors
    C) omission errors
    D) compliance errors

23. Which is NOT a part of a syringe?
    A) tip
    B) plunger
    C) lumen
    D) barrel

24. Third-party payers
    A) are contracted by insurance companies to collect payments and debts from patients.
    B) are the patients.
    C) are the insurance companies.
    D) are used by the health insurance company to manage prescription drug benefits.

25. Which incident helped to pass the Food, Drug, and Cosmetic Act of 1938?
    A) the International Opium Convention
    B) the Sulfanilamide Tragedy
    C) the Thalidomide Tragedy
    D) the hundreds of deaths of children under the age of five as a result of ingesting drugs and household chemicals

26. Deteriorated drug errors are

   A) due to incorrectly monitored drugs that require specific laboratory values for medication and dose selections.

   B) caused by using expired drugs or drugs whose chemical or physical potency and integrity has somehow been compromised.

   C) made typically by nurses in drug administration. Errors are due to failure to properly follow protocols, performance deficit, and lack of knowledge.

   D) when the prescribed dose is not administered at the correct time.

27. Which is NOT a type of medication order?

   A) scheduled

   B) as needed (PRN)

   C) blood testing

   D) controlled substance

28. Multiply $\frac{4}{5} \times \frac{7}{8}$. What is the answer in the lowest possible terms?

   A) $\frac{28}{40}$

   B) $\frac{4}{20}$

   C) $\frac{14}{20}$

   D) $\frac{7}{10}$

29. Which digestive enzymes do NOT pass from the exocrine tissue of the pancreas to the small intestine?

   A) pancreatic amylase

   B) trypsin

   C) pancreatic lipase

   D) insulin

30. What can workers do in the clean room?

   A) garb

   B) generate labels

   C) prepare CSPs

   D) wash hands

31. The US Pharmacopeia (USP) was developed under which act?

   A) the Food, Drug, and Cosmetic Act of 1938

   B) the Controlled Substance Act

   C) the Orphan Drug Act

   D) the Pure Food and Drug Act of 1906

32. Which drug is considered a SALAD drug?

   A) Alprazolam

   B) Meloxicam

   C) Hydrochlorothiazide

   D) Clomiphene

33. Drug duplication

   A) is when a drug is prescribed that shares an active ingredient with a medication a patient is already taking.

   B) is when drugs are in the same drug class or have the same function in the body.

   C) is when drugs contain more than one active ingredient to treat separate conditions.

   D) could be anything that causes restrictions on the patient.

34. How many tablespoonsful are in 2 ounces?

   A) 4 tablespoonsful

   B) 2 tablespoonsful

   C) 1 tablespoonful

   D) 3 tablespoonsful

35. Which act or amendment required that the phrase, "Caution: Federal Law Prohibits Dispensing without a Prescription" be placed on prescription labeling?

   A) the Food, Drug, and Cosmetic Act of 1938

   B) the Kefauver-Harris Amendment of 1962

   C) the Durham-Humphrey Amendment of 1951

   D) the Controlled Substance Act

36. Which is NOT a side effect of montelukast?

   A) diarrhea

   B) headache

   C) flu symptoms

   D) sore throat

37. POS plans

   A) still require an in-network primary care physician; however a patient can get out-of-network services at a higher cost.

   B) usually limit coverage to care from in-network doctors and specialists for a fixed annual fee and/or copayment for services rendered.

   C) allow patients to see any in-network physician or specialist without needing a prior authorization, although they need to meet annual deductibles.

   D) provide coverage to people who are injured on the job.

38. How often should the weights on a class A balance be calibrated?

   A) every six months

   B) every other year

   C) three times a year

   D) annually

39. The prefix *cirrh–* means

   A) green.

   B) blue.

   C) red.

   D) yellow.

40. What is a potential error if there is a mix-up between the SALAD drugs clonidine and Klonopin?

   A) renal failure, respiratory arrest, and even death

   B) loss of seizure control, hypotension, or other serious consequences

   C) hypoglycemia or poor diabetes control

   D) inability to manage pain, abnormal psychiatric symptoms, or other serious consequences

41. Which act outlines the process for drug companies to file an abbreviated new drug application (ANDA)?

   A) the Drug Price Competition and Patent Term Restoration Act of 1984

   B) the Health Insurance Portability and Accountability Act (HIPAA) of 1996

   C) the Patient Protection and Affordable Care Act of 2010

   D) the Drug Listing Act

42. Which of the following is NOT true about refill authorizations?

   A) They are called in by the patient.

   B) They may not be approved for controlled substances due to federal and state laws.

   C) Further refills are called in by the doctor.

   D) They may not be approved for short-term conditions (e.g., cough medicines).

43. How is MMMDCVI written in arabic numerals?

   A) 3,606
   B) 3,666
   C) 366
   D) 1,306

44. The suffix –raxole refers to which drug class?

   A) opioid narcotics
   B) proton pump inhibitors
   C) ACE inhibitors
   D) benzodiazepines

45. In hospitals, how many people die annually from medication errors?

   A) 100,000
   B) 400,000
   C) 300,000
   D) 500,000

46. Which is an abbreviation used for a nursing unit in the hospital?

   A) ATC
   B) ENDO
   C) STAT
   D) TID

47. How many digits does an NDC number consist of?

   A) nine
   B) ten
   C) twelve
   D) eight

48. With TRICARE, which plan is an HMO?

   A) Standard
   B) Extra
   C) Prime
   D) Basic

49. Which is NOT a microorganism that can be transmitted during sterile compounding?

   A) fungi
   B) amoeba
   C) bacteria
   D) virus

50. Online adjudication

   A) is the process of sending a claim to the third-party payer for reimbursement.
   B) is the deductible.
   C) refers to billing the third party for goods and services rendered.
   D) is the compensation given to the pharmacy after collection of the patient's copay or deductible.

51. Which of the following is $\frac{1}{4}$ grain equivalent to?

   A) 1 mgs
   B) 15 mgs
   C) 30 mgs
   D) 60 mgs

52. Which of the following is NOT a cause of high cholesterol?

   A) poor diet
   B) smoking
   C) genetic factors
   D) exercise

53. Most medication errors occur because of all of the following EXCEPT

   A) education and training.
   B) failure to follow procedures.
   C) poor performance.
   D) miscommunication.

54. If a patient has a history of drug abuse, pharmacists do all of the following EXCEPT

A) monitor controlled medications.

B) put restrictions on controlled medications.

C) make sure the patient is complying with the directions.

D) tell a family member to monitor the patient's use of the medication.

55. How many mgs are equivalent to 5.8 g?

A) 58 mgs

B) 0.58 mgs

C) 580 mgs

D) 5,800 mgs

56. The first five digits of the NDC number refer to the

A) labeler.

B) drug.

C) package.

D) pharmacy.

57. Medication errors that occur because of metabolism problems in patients are due to

A) social causes.

B) calculation errors.

C) abbreviation errors.

D) physiological make up.

58. Which form of hepatitis cannot spread by sexual contact?

A) Hepatitis A

B) Hepatitis B

C) Hepatitis C

D) Hepatitis cannot be transmitted sexually.

59. NDC numbers were implemented under which act?

A) the Orphan Drug Act

B) the FDA Modernization Act

C) the Medicare Modernization Act

D) the Drug Listing Act of 1972

60. Which is a part of Medicare Part A?

A) Used for doctor's services

B) Covers Medicare Advantage Plans

C) Covers prescription drugs

D) Used for inpatient stays

61. The sig code QID is defined as

A) every day.

B) every other day.

C) four times daily.

D) three times daily.

62. Which is NOT a part of the clean room of the pharmacy?

A) faucet

B) laminar airflow workbench

C) barrier isolators

D) buffer area

63. Which is NOT a true statement in regards to expired medications?

A) Drugs expiring within 1 month must be pulled from the shelves.

B) If a drug's expiration date states 6/19, the drug is good until 6/30/2019.

C) Stock bottles should be marked accordingly to alert staff that the medication is expiring within the next 3 months.

D) Expired medications must be stored in a designated area away from regular stock.

64. Another word for co-insurance is:

   A) Deductible

   B) Fee-for-service

   C) Retrospective payment

   D) Dispensing fee

65. What is a part of a syringe needle?

   A) filter

   B) adaptor

   C) shaft

   D) tip

66. In the expression $\frac{3}{8} + \frac{2}{5}$, what is the lowest common denominator?

   A) 20

   B) 40

   C) 4

   D) 8

67. The prefix *peri–* means

   A) inner.

   B) around.

   C) out.

   D) under.

68. Which medical device class of the Medical Device Amendment of 1976 referred to general controlled devices with low risks to humans?

   A) Class IV

   B) Class II

   C) Class I

   D) Class III

69. Which of the following groups is most commonly affected by calculation errors?

   A) the elderly

   B) women

   C) children

   D) men

70. Which agency has the complete authority to enforce the Resource Conservation and Recovery Act of 1976?

   A) FDA

   B) DEA

   C) CIA

   D) EPA

71. If a healthcare provider is unable to make an outpatient comply with directions for the use of a prescription drug, this error is due to _____.

   A) physiological make up

   B) an abbreviation error

   C) a calculation error

   D) social causes

72. Which dosage is NOT presented on a dose response curve in regards to clinical trials?

   A) TD50

   B) LD50

   C) RD50

   D) ED50

73. Which DAW means the prescriber is NOT allowing generic substitution?

   A) 5

   B) 8

   C) 1

   D) 3

74. Which is NOT an incidence of noncompliance in regards to MTM?

   A) A patient takes another person's medication to avoid copays.

   B) The patient's doctor discontinued the medication.

   C) The patient is skipping doses.

   D) A patient has stopped taking his or her medication altogether.

75. Child doses are calculated by the child's

    A) weight.

    B) height.

    C) age.

    D) grade.

76. What is NOT necessary in garbing up?

    A) shoe covers

    B) mask

    C) gloves

    D) to wash the face

77. How many drams are in 4 ounces?

    A) 16 drams

    B) 8 drams

    C) 32 drams

    D) 4 drams

78. Which of the following does the drug succinylcholine treat?

    A) blood pressure

    B) pain

    C) anesthesia

    D) It is an immunosuppressant.

79. About what percentage of the United States population has insurance?

    A) 99%

    B) 75%

    C) 84%

    D) 63%

80. 480 mL is equivalent to how many pints?

    A) 2 pints

    B) 4 pints

    C) $\frac{1}{2}$ pint

    D) 1 pint

81. Which drug is considered a high-alert medication?

    A) Metronidazole

    B) potassium chloride injections

    C) Ketorolac

    D) Lisinopril

82. Arteries

    A) transfer blood away from the heart.

    B) transfer blood to the heart.

    C) are small vessels found in the tissue.

    D) are thin walled, valved structures that carry lymph.

83. What is the main purpose of MTM?

    A) to reduce costs for insurance companies

    B) to increase calls to doctors to obtain refills

    C) to advise patients of delivery or mail-order options

    D) to improve patient compliance

84. Orphan drugs are

    A) drugs that cure diseases.

    B) prescribed for common diseases and conditions.

    C) pharmaceuticals that are developed specifically for rare diseases.

    D) drugs anyone can qualify to use.

85. Hypertension occurs when the blood pressure reading is over

    A) 120/80.

    B) 100/70.

    C) 140/90.

    D) 110/60.

86. What information is NOT found in a compounding log?

   A) physician's name

   B) lot number

   C) pharmacist's initials

   D) beyond-use date

87. Benztropine is an

   A) Alzheimer's disease medication.

   B) anti-tremor medication.

   C) anti-anxiety medication.

   D) anti-depressant medication.

88. Which of the following is NOT a part of the patient's profile?

   A) Allergy information

   B) Spouse's name

   C) Patient's date of birth

   D) Insurance information

89. All of these are strategies used to differentiate SALAD drugs from regular stock EXCEPT

   A) avoiding the risk by not stocking SALAD drugs in the pharmacy.

   B) using Tallman lettering.

   C) color-coding.

   D) stocking SALAD drugs in a different area in the pharmacy, away from the regular stock.

90. How many mL are in 2 teaspoonsful?

   A) 15 mL

   B) 5 mL

   C) 10 mL

   D) 20 mL

1. A) Incorrect. The suffix *–olol* refers to beta blockers.

    B) Incorrect. The suffix *–pril* refers to ACE inhibitors.

    C) Correct. The suffix *–tidine* is used for histamine-2 blockers.

    D) Incorrect. The suffix *–artan* is used for angiotensin 2 receptor blockers.

2. A) Incorrect. A class A balance does not weigh this much.

    B) Correct. The weight limit of a class A balance is 120 mg.

    C) Incorrect. Class A balances can weigh 100 mg, but they may weigh even more.

    D) Incorrect. Class A balances weigh far less than 360 mg.

3. A) Incorrect. Using cc instead of mL can be an abbreviation error.

    B) Incorrect. Using apothecary units instead of metric units can be an abbreviation error.

    C) Correct. Using STAT instead of as soon as possible is acceptable.

    D) Incorrect. Using MS in an unclear manner may be an abbreviation error.

4. **A) Correct.** Barcode administration technology reduces medication errors by using a barcode on the patient's label that matches the inpatient's bar code on their wristband to verify the correct patient is being scanned before medication is administered.

    B) Incorrect. Web-based compliance and disease management tracking systems helps to track patient's compliance with taking maintenance medications and tracking disease management through software systems connected to physician's offices, hospitals, and pharmacies.

    C) Incorrect. Unit-dose repacking systems are used to unit dose medications in stock bottles in the centralized pharmacy.

    D) IV and TPN compounding devices are automatic pumping systems that can compound several sterile ingredients into a finished solution dispensed in a single patient bag without being manually touched by the technician.

5. A) Incorrect. Ondansetron is not used for pain.

    B) Incorrect. Ondansetron is not used to treat diabetes.

    C) Incorrect. Ondansetron does not treat stomach acid.

    D) Correct. Ondansetron is used for nausea.

6. A) Incorrect. Leukemia is a disease of the immune system.

    B) Incorrect. Cystitis is a disease of the urinary system.

    C) Incorrect. Angina affects the circulatory system.

    D) Correct. Osteoarthritis is a musculoskeletal condition.

7. A) Incorrect. Less than 3 million medication errors occur in the United States each year.

    B) Incorrect. There are not 5 million medication errors in the United States each year.

    C) Correct. Nearly 1.5 million medication errors occur each year.

    D) Incorrect. Less than 2.5 million medication errors occur in the United States each year.

8. A) Incorrect. The PCN number is used by PBMs for network benefit routing and may change depending on what benefit is being billed.

    B) Correct. The BIN number directs the claim to the correct third-party provider.

    C) Incorrect. The group number directs the claim to specific insurance benefits for that group.

    D) Incorrect. The patient's date of birth is used as an identification tool; an insurance card displays the dates of birth for each person covered next to his or her name.

9. **B)**

Break up the arabic number:

2014 = 2000 + 10 + 4

Plug in the roman numeral values.

2000 = MM, 10 = X, 4 = IV (5 − 1), since I is before V.

= MMXIV

10. A) Incorrect. The root word *hepat/o* refers to the liver.

   B) **Correct.** The root word *lapar/o* refers to the abdomen.

   C) Incorrect. The root word *hist/o* refers to body tissue.

   D) Incorrect. The root words *mamm/o* or *mast/o* refer to the breast.

11. A) Incorrect. The patient's name is required on a non-control hard copy.

   B) **Correct.** Although it is normally pre-printed on the hard copy, the DEA number is not required on a non-control.

   C) Incorrect. The patient's phone number must be included on a non-control hard copy.

   D) Incorrect. A non-control hard copy must display the prescriber's name.

12. **A)** **Correct.** Salmeterol prevents asthma attacks and bronchospasms.

   B) Incorrect. Salmeterol does not lower fevers or treat inflammation.

   C) Incorrect. Salmeterol is not used to treat autoimmune disorders.

   D) Incorrect. Salmeterol is not an estrogen modulator.

13. **A)** **Correct.** USB chapter 795 discusses the standards required for non-sterile compounding.

   B) Incorrect. There is no USB 799.

   C) Incorrect. USB chapter 797 addresses sterile compounding.

   D) Incorrect. USB chapter 796 does not reference non-sterile compounding.

14. **A)**

Find equivalent fractions with the common denominator 40.

$\frac{3}{8} = \frac{15}{40}, \frac{2}{5} = \frac{16}{40}$

Add the numerators of the fractions and leave the denominator. This fraction cannot be reduced.

$\frac{3}{8} + \frac{2}{5} = \frac{15}{40} + \frac{16}{40} = \mathbf{\frac{31}{40}}$

15. **A)** **Correct.** Harvey Wiley helped to pass the Pure Food and Drug Act of 1906.

   B) Incorrect. The Food, Drug, and Cosmetic Act of 1938 was separate from the Pure Food and Drug Act.

   C) Incorrect. Harvey Wiley did not lead efforts to pass the Poison Prevention Packaging Act.

   D) Incorrect. Harvey Wiley was not a driver of the Harrison Narcotics Tax Act of 1914.

16. A) Incorrect. The suffix *–tomy* refers to an incision.

   B) Incorrect. The suffix *–plasia* refers to a formation.

   C) Incorrect. The suffix *–osis* refers to an abnormal condition.

   D) **Correct.** The suffix *–stomy* refers to an artificial opening.

17. A) Incorrect. POS plans are managed care plans

   B) Incorrect. HMOs are managed care plans.

   C) Incorrect. PPOs are managed care plans.

   D) **Correct.** PAPs are for self-pay patients.

18. A) Incorrect. Medication errors are a primary cause of preventable death and injuries, but they are not the leading one.

   B) Incorrect. Medication errors are not the fifth leading cause of preventable death and injuries.

C)   Incorrect. Medication errors are not the fourth leading cause of preventable death and injuries.

D)   **Correct.** Medication errors are the third leading cause of preventable death and injuries in the United States.

19.   **C)**

Set up a proportion with mL on top and L on bottom. Recall that 1000 mL = 1 L.

$$\frac{1000 \text{ mL}}{1 \text{ L}} = \frac{3600 \text{ mL}}{x \text{ L}}$$

Cross-multiply and solve for x.

$1000x = 3600$

$x = \textbf{3.6 L}$

Note: This can also be solved using Dimensional Analysis, multiplying by conversion ratios to cancel out units until finding the needed units. Here, ratios are set up so that unwanted units cross out on top and bottom:

$$3600 \text{ mL} \times \frac{1 \text{ L}}{1000 \text{ mL}} = 3.6 \text{ L}$$

20.   **A)**   **Correct.** Pharmacodynamics is how the action, effect, and breakdown of drugs happens in the body.

B)   Incorrect. The difference in quantity of medication between the effective dose and the amount that causes adverse side effects is called the therapeutic window.

C)   Incorrect. Bioequivalence is when two drugs have the same bioavailability.

D)   Incorrect. Pharmacodynamics does not address what happens if a patient decides not to take a drug the physician prescribes.

21.   **A)**   **Correct.** The FDA was formed in 1906.

B)   Incorrect. The FDA did not form in 1938.

C)   Incorrect. The US Department of Agriculture was formed in 1862.

D)   Incorrect. The Bureau of Chemistry was formed in 1901.

22.   A)   Incorrect. Wrong dosage form errors occur when the prescribed route of administration of the drug is incorrect.

B)   Incorrect. Improper dose errors occur when the patient receives a lesser dose, a higher dose, or extra doses of the drug than what was prescribed.

C)   **Correct.** Omission errors occur when the prescribed dose is not administered as ordered.

D)   Incorrect. Compliance errors occur when the patient does not take the drug the way the doctor prescribes it.

23.   A)   Incorrect. The tip is where the needle is attached.

B)   Incorrect. The plunger is the cylinder that inserts into the barrel of the syringe.

C)   **Correct.** The lumen is part of the syringe needle.

D)   Incorrect. The barrel is the part that holds the medication and displays the calibrations.

24.   A)   **Correct.** Third-party payers are contracted by insurance companies to collect payments and debts from patients.

B)   Incorrect. Patients are first-party payers.

C)   Incorrect. Insurance companies are second-party payers.

D)   Incorrect. PBMs manage prescription drug benefits for health insurance companies.

25.   A)   Incorrect. The Harrison Narcotics Tax Act of 1914 was passed because of the International Opium Convention.

B)   **Correct.** The Food, Drug and Cosmetic Act of 1938 was passed because of the Sulfanilamide tragedy.

C)   Incorrect. The Kefauver-Harris Amendment of 1962 was passed because of the Thalidomide Tragedy.

D)   Incorrect. The Poison Prevention Packaging Act was passed because of the hundreds of deaths of children under the age of five as a result of ingesting drugs and household chemicals.

26.   A)   Incorrect. Monitoring errors are due to incorrectly monitored drugs that require specific laboratory values for medication and dose selections.

B) **Correct.** Deteriorated drug errors are caused by using expired drugs or drugs whose chemical or physical potency and integrity has somehow been compromised.

C. Incorrect. These situations are called wrong administration technique errors.

D.) Incorrect. These instances are wrong time errors.

27. A) Incorrect. Scheduled medication orders are for those medications given around the clock.

B) Incorrect. PRN is a type of medication order; these medications are provided on an as-needed basis.

C) **Correct.** Blood testing is not a type of medication order.

D) Incorrect. Medication orders include controlled substances.

28. **D)**

Multiply numerators across and denominators across.

$$\frac{4}{5} \times \frac{7}{8} = \frac{4 \times 7}{5 \times 8} = \frac{28}{40}$$

Reduce (simplify) answer to simplest terms.

$$\frac{28}{40} = \frac{7 \times 4}{10 \times 4} = \frac{7}{10}$$

29. A) Incorrect. Pancreatic amylase is a digestive enzyme that passes to the small intestine.

B) Incorrect. Trypsin is a digestive enzyme that passes to the small intestine.

C) Incorrect. Pancreatic lipase is a digestive enzyme that passes to the small intestine.

D) **Correct.** Insulin is not a digestive enzyme.

30. A) Incorrect. Workers may only garb in the anteroom.

B) Incorrect. No paper is permitted in the clean room, so labels must be generated in the anteroom.

C) **Correct.** CSPs are prepared in the sterile room under the laminar airflow hood.

D) Incorrect. Workers can use an antibacterial solution to sterilize their

hands in the clean room, but aseptic handwashing is done at the faucet in the anteroom.

31. **A)** **Correct.** The Food, Drug and Cosmetic Act of 1938 developed the USP.

B) Incorrect. The Controlled Substance Act controls the manufacture, importation, possession, use, and distribution of certain controlled substances.

C) Incorrect. The Orphan Drug Act supports the development drugs to treat rare, or orphan, diseases.

D) Incorrect. The Pure Food and Drug Act of 1906 required manufacturers to properly label a drug with truthful information.

32. A) Incorrect. Alprazolam is not a SALAD drug.

B) Incorrect. Meloxicam is not considered a SALAD drug.

C) Incorrect. Hydrochlorothiazide is not considered a SALAD drug.

D) **Correct.** Clomiphene is a SALAD drug.

33. **A)** **Correct.** Drug duplications happen if a patient is prescribed a new drug that contains an active ingredient shared by a medication he or she already takes.

B) Incorrect. Therapeutic duplication refers to situations when drugs are in the same drug class or have the same function in the body.

C) Incorrect. Drugs have more than one active ingredient in them that are used for separate conditions are called combination drugs.

D) Incorrect. Special conditions could be anything that causes restrictions on the patient.

34. **A)**

Set up a proportion with ounces on top and tablespoons on the bottom. Recall that $\frac{1}{2}$ fl.ounce = 1 tablespoon.

$$\frac{\frac{1}{2} \text{ fl.ounce}}{1 \text{ tablespoon}} = \frac{2 \text{ fl.ounce}}{x \text{ tablespoons}}$$

Cross-multiply and solve for x.

$$\frac{1}{2}x = 2$$

x = **4 tablespoonsful**

Note: This can also be solved using Dimensional Analysis, multiplying by conversion ratios to cancel out units until finding the needed units:

$$2 \text{ fl.ounces} \times \frac{1 \text{ tablespoon}}{\frac{1}{2} \text{ fl.ounce}} = 4 \text{ tablespoonsful}$$

35. A) Incorrect. The Food, Drug, and Cosmetic Act of 1938 required a ban on false claims, required package inserts with directions to be included with products, and required exact labeling on the product.

   B) Incorrect. The Kefauver-Harris Amendment gave the FDA the authority to approve a manufacturer's marketing application before the drug was to become available for consumer or commercial use.

   C) **Correct.** The Durham-Humphrey Amendment required the phrase, "Caution: Federal Law Prohibits Dispensing without a Prescription" be placed on prescription labeling.

   D) Incorrect. The Controlled Substance Act controls the manufacture, importation, possession, use, and distribution of certain controlled substances.

36. **A)** **Correct.** Diarrhea is not a side effect of montelukast.

   B) Incorrect. Headaches are a side effect of montelukast.

   C) Incorrect. Flu symptoms are a possible side effect of montelukast.

   D) Incorrect. One side effect of montelukast is a sore throat.

37. **A)** **Correct.** POS plans still require an in-network primary care physician, but a patient can get out-of-network services at a higher cost.

   B) Incorrect. HMO plans usually limit coverage to care from in-network doctors and specialists for a fixed annual fee and/or copayment for services rendered.

   C) Incorrect. PPO plans allow patients to see any in-network physician or specialist without needing a prior authorization, although they need to meet annual deductibles.

   D) Incorrect: Worker's Compensation provides coverage to people injured on the job.

38. A) Incorrect. Class A balances are not calibrated twice a year.

   B) Incorrect. Class A balances require more frequent upkeep.

   C) Incorrect. Class A balances do not need to be calibrated this often.

   D) **Correct.** Class A balances must be calibrated and certified every year.

39. A) Incorrect. The prefix *chlor–* means green.

   B) Incorrect. The prefix *cyan–* refers to blue.

   C) Incorrect. The prefix *eryth–* refers to red.

   D) **Correct.** The prefix *cirrh–* means yellow.

40. A) Incorrect. Errors in amphotericin B products could result in renal failure, respiratory arrest, and even death.

   B) **Correct.** Confusing clonidine and Klonopin may result in loss of seizure control, hypotension, or other serious consequences

   C) Incorrect. Mixing up different forms of insulin may result in hypoglycemia or poor diabetes control.

   D) Incorrect. Confusing the SALAD drugs tramadol, trazodone, and toradol may result in an inability to manage pain, abnormal psychiatric symptoms, or other serious consequences.

41. **A)** **Correct.** The Drug Price Competition and Patent Term Restoration Act of 1984 outlines the process for drug companies to file an abbreviated new drug application (ANDA).

   B) Incorrect. The Health Insurance Portability and Accountability Act (HIPAA) of 1996 established protected health information and safeguards patient privacy.

   C) Incorrect. The Patient Protection and Affordable Care Act of 2010 required individuals to have health insurance and required insurance companies to cover all individuals with new minimum standards in order to increase the quality and affordability of healthcare.

D) Incorrect. The Drug Listing Act implemented the national drug code number (NDC).

42. **A) Correct.** The doctor must approve a refill authorization.

B) Incorrect. Authorizations may not be approved for controlled substances due to federal or state laws.

C) Incorrect. Refill authorizations are called in by the doctor.

D) Incorrect. Refill authorizations may not be approved for short-term conditions.

43. **A)**
Break up the roman numeral.
MMMDCVI = MMM + D + C + V + I
Plug in the arabic numeral values.
MMMDCVI = 3000 + 500 + 100 + 5 + 1
= 3,606

44. A) Incorrect. The suffix –codone refers to opioid narcotics.

B) Correct. The suffix –praxole refers to proton pump inhibitors.

C) Incorrect. The suffix –pril refers to ACE inhibitors.

D) Incorrect. The suffix –pam refers to benzodiazepines.

45. A) Incorrect. Over 100,000 people die in hospitals from medication errors every year.

B) Correct. Every year, 400,000 people die in hospitals due to medication errors alone.

C) Incorrect. More than 300,000 people die annually in hospitals from medication errors.

D) Incorrect. Less than 500,000 people die each year in hospitals from medication errors.

46. A) Incorrect. ATC means around the clock.

B) Correct. ENDO means endoscopy.

C) Incorrect. STAT means right away.

D) Incorrect. TID stands for three times daily.

47. A) Incorrect. An NDC number contains more than nine digits.

B) Correct. NDC numbers contain ten digits.

C) Incorrect. NDC numbers do not contain twelve digits.

D) Incorrect. NDC numbers contain more than eight digits.

48. A) Incorrect. Standard is a fee-for-service cost-sharing plan.

B) Correct. Extra is an HMO plan.

C) Incorrect. Prime is a PPO with a POS option.

D) Incorrect. Basic is not a plan at all under TRICARE.

49. A) Incorrect. Fungi can be transmitted during sterile compounding and can cause yeast and fungal infections in patients.

B) Correct. Amoebas are not found in pharmacy environments.

C) Incorrect. Bacteria can be transmitted by sterile compounding and cause pyrogens to enter the bloodstream if the technician does not comply with aseptic technique.

D) Incorrect. Viruses can be transmitted if the technician does not comply with aseptic technique.

50. A) Incorrect. Claim submission is the process of sending a claim to the third-party payer for reimbursement.

B) Incorrect. Co-insurance is the deductible.

C) Correct. Online adjudication is billing a third party for goods and services rendered.

D) Incorrect. Reimbursement is the compensation given to the pharmacy after collection of the patient's copay or deductible.

51. B)

Set up a proportion with grains on top and mg on the bottom. Recall that 1 grain ≈ 60 – 65 mg. Use 62 mg.

$$\frac{1 \text{ grain}}{62 \text{ mg}} = \frac{\frac{1}{4} \text{ grain}}{x \text{ mg}}$$

Cross-multiply and solve for x.

$$x = 62 \times \frac{1}{4}$$

$$x \approx \textbf{15 mgs}$$

Note: This can also be solved using Dimensional Analysis, multiplying by conversion ratios to cancel out units until finding the needed units:

$$\frac{1}{4} \text{ grain} \times \frac{62 \text{ mg}}{1 \text{ grain}} \approx 15 \text{ mgs}$$

52. A) Incorrect. Poor diet can cause high cholesterol.

B) Incorrect. Smoking is a cause of high cholesterol.

C) Incorrect. Genetic factors may cause high cholesterol.

D) Correct. Exercise is not a cause of high cholesterol.

53. A) Correct. Education and training prevent medication errors.

B) Incorrect. Failure to follow procedures can cause medication errors.

C) Incorrect. Poor performance is one cause of medication errors.

D) Incorrect. Many medication errors are caused by miscommunication.

54. A) Incorrect. The pharmacist may monitor the medication.

B) Incorrect. The pharmacist may put restrictions on the medication.

C) Incorrect. The pharmacist may make sure the patient is complying with the directions for use.

D) Correct. The pharmacist would be violating HIPAA if she or he told a family member to monitor the patient without the patient's permission.

55. D)

Set up a proportion with g on top and mg on bottom. Use the fact that 1 g = 1000 mg.

$$\frac{1 \text{ g}}{1000 \text{ mg}} = \frac{5.8 \text{ g}}{x \text{ mg}}$$

Cross-multiply and solve for x.

$$x = \textbf{5800 mgs}$$

56. A) Correct. The first five digits refer to the labeler code.

B) Incorrect. The second group of numbers refers to the drug code.

C) Incorrect. The last two digits refer to the package code.

D) Incorrect. The pharmacy is not identified on the package code.

57. A) Incorrect. Social causes of medication errors are not due to metabolism problems in patients.

B) Incorrect. Calculation errors are not due to metabolism problems in patients.

C) Incorrect. Abbreviation errors are not due to metabolism problems in patients.

D) Correct. Physiological make up causes medication errors because of metabolism problems in patients.

58. A) Correct. Hepatitis A is spread by contamination of food and water.

B) Incorrect. Hepatitis B can be spread by sexual contact.

C) Incorrect. Hepatitis C can be spread by sexual contact.

D) Incorrect. Hepatitis B and C can be transmitted through sexual contact.

59. A) Incorrect. The Orphan Drug Act did not implement NDC numbers.

B) Incorrect. The FDA Modernization Act did not implement NDC numbers.

C) Incorrect. The Medicare Modernization Act did not implement NDC numbers.

D) Correct. The Drug Listing Act of 1972 implemented NDC numbers.

60. A) Incorrect. Medicare Part A is not used for doctor's services.

B) Incorrect. Medicare Part A does not cover Medicare Advantage Plans.

C) Incorrect. Medicare Part A does not cover prescription drugs.

D) Correct. Medicare Part A is used for inpatient stays.

61.
A) Incorrect. QD is the sig code for every day.
B) Incorrect. The sig code for every other day is QOD.
C) Correct. QID means four times daily.
D) Incorrect. TID means three times daily.

62.
A) Correct. The faucet is located in the anteroom.
B) Incorrect. The laminar airflow workbench is where the technician prepares CSPs in the clean room.
C) Incorrect. Technicians use barrier isolators in the clean room as another safeguard against contamination so they can prepare CSPs in an aseptic box under the hood.
D) Incorrect. The buffer area is the area immediately next to the laminar airflow hood in the clean room.

63.
A) Incorrect. Drugs expiring within 1 month must be pulled from the shelves.
B) Correct. If a drug's expiration date states 6/19, the drug will indeed expire on 6/30/2019.
C) Incorrect. It is true that stock bottles should be marked accordingly to alert staff that the medication is expiring within the next 3 months.
D) Incorrect. Expired medications must be stored in a designated area away from regular stock.

64.
A) Correct. Another word for co-insurance is deductible.
B) Incorrect. Fee-for-service is not a deductible.
C) Incorrect. Retrospective payment is not a deductible.
D) Incorrect. Dispensing fee is not a deductible.

65.
A) Incorrect. A filter removes unwanted particles from a solution.
B) Incorrect. An adaptor is an attachment used for transferring medication from an IV bag to a vial (and vice versa).
C) Correct. The shaft is the long, narrow, hollow point of the needle.

D) Incorrect. The tip is a part of the syringe, not the needle. The needle is attached to the syringe at the tip.

66. B)
The least common denominator is the least common multiple of 8 and 5.
5: 5, 10, 15, 20, 25, 30, 35, **40**
8: 8, 16, 24, 32, **40**

67.
A) Incorrect. The prefix *endo–* means inner.
B) Correct. The prefix *peri–* means around.
C) Incorrect. The prefix *exo–* means out.
D) Incorrect. The prefix *sub–* means under.

68.
A) Incorrect. There is no Class IV listed in the Medical Device Amendment of 1976.
B) Incorrect. Class II devices are performance standard devices that are considered to pose moderate risks for human use.
C) Correct. Class I devices are general controlled devices that are low risk for human use.
D) Incorrect. Class III devices require premarket approval applications that are the equivalent to a new drug application.

69.
A) Incorrect. The elderly are not the most commonly population affected by calculation errors.
B) Incorrect. Women are not the group most commonly affected by calculation errors.
C) Correct. Children are most commonly affected by calculation errors.
D) Incorrect. Men are not as commonly affected by calculation errors as children are.

70.
A) Incorrect. The FDA does not have the complete authority to enforce the Resource Conservation and Recovery Act of 1976.
B) Incorrect. The DEA does not have the complete authority to enforce the

Resource Conservation and Recovery Act of 1976.

C) Incorrect. The CIA is not authorized to enforce the Resource Conservation and Recovery Act of 1976 and is not involved in such work.

D) Correct. The EPA has the complete authority to enforce the Resource Conservation and Recovery Act of · 1976.

71. A) Incorrect. Medication error due to patient noncompliance with directions for medication use is not a result of the patient's physiological make up.

B) Incorrect. An abbreviation error would not result in a medication error due to intentional patient noncompliance with directions for medication use.

C) Incorrect. A calculation error would not result in a medication error due to intentional patient noncompliance with directions for medication use.

D) Correct. Patient noncompliance with directions for medication use is a medication error due to social causes.

72. A) Incorrect. TD50 is a dosage presented on a dose response curve.

B) Incorrect. LD50 is a dosage found on a dose response curve.

C) Correct. There is no RD50 dose on a dose response curve.

D) Incorrect. ED50 is a dosage presented on a dose response curve.

73. A) Incorrect. DAW 5 means that a brand name medication is dispensed at generic price. Substitution is allowed.

B) Incorrect. DAW 8 means the generic version of a drug is not available. Substitution is allowed.

C) Correct. DAW 1 indicates that substitutions are not allowed by the prescriber. This is used when the doctor deems the brand medication is medically necessary, and substitution is not allowed.

D) Incorrect. DAW 3 indicates that the pharmacist selected the brand name although substitution is allowed.

74. A) Incorrect. Taking another person's medication to avoid copays is being noncompliant.

B) Correct. If the patient is not taking a medication because the doctor discontinued the medication, the patient is still compliant.

C) Incorrect. Skipping doses means a patient is noncompliant.

D) Incorrect. A patient who stops taking medication altogether without the doctor's approval is noncompliant.

75. **A) Correct.** Child doses are calculated by weight and BSA.

B) Incorrect. Child doses are not calculated by height.

C) Incorrect. A child's age does not determine medication dosage.

D) Incorrect. A child's grade has no bearing on medication.

76. A) Incorrect. Shoe covers are required; they are the first PPE put on when garbing up.

B) Incorrect. Technicians use masks to avoid contaminating the clean room with body particulates.

C) Incorrect. Gloves are required in the clean room, so they are an important part of garbing up.

D) Correct. Although technicians and other workers should wear minimal or no make up in the clean room, they are not required to wash their faces while garbing up.

77. **C)**

Set up a proportion with ounces on top and drams on bottom. Recall that 1 fl.ounce = 8 drams.

$$\frac{1 \text{ fl.ounce}}{8 \text{ drams}} = \frac{4 \text{ fl.ounce}}{x \text{ drams}}$$

Cross-multiply and solve for x.

$x = $ **32 drams**

Note: This can also be solved using Dimensional Analysis, multiplying by conversion ratios to cancel out units until finding the needed units:

4 fl.ounces $\times \frac{8 \text{ drams}}{1 \text{ fl.ounce}} = 32$ drams

78.
A) Incorrect. Succinylcholine is not used to treat blood pressure.

B) Incorrect. Succinylcholine is not used for pain.

C) Correct. Succinylcholine is used as anesthesia and is a paralytic agent.

D) Incorrect. Succinylcholine is not an immunosuppressant.

79.
A) Incorrect. While more Americans than ever before are insured, this number is far too high.

B) Incorrect. More than 75% of Americans are insured, so this number is incorrect.

C) Correct. As of 2016, about 84% of Americans are insured.

D) Incorrect. This number is too low and therefore incorrect.

80. D)

Set up a proportion with mL on top and pints on the bottom. Recall that 480 mL = 1 pint.

$$\frac{480 \text{ mL}}{1 \text{ pint}} = \frac{480 \text{ mL}}{x \text{ pints}}$$

Cross-multiply and solve for x.

$$480x = 480$$

$$x = 1 \text{ pint}$$

Note: This can also be solved using Dimensional Analysis, multiplying by conversion ratios to cancel out units until finding the needed units:

$$480 \text{ mL} \times \frac{1 \text{ pint}}{480 \text{ mL}} = 1 \text{ pint}$$

81.
A) Incorrect. Metronidazole is not considered a high-alert medication.

B) Correct. Potassium chloride injections are considered high-alert.

C) Incorrect. Ketorolac is not high-alert medication.

D) Incorrect. Lisinopril is not considered a high-alert medication.

82.
A) Correct. Arteries carry blood away from the heart.

B) Incorrect. Veins carry blood to the heart.

C) Incorrect. Capillaries are the small vessels in tissue.

D) Incorrect. Thin-walled, valved structures that carry lymph are called lymph vessels.

83.
A) Incorrect. MTM is not necessarily intended to reduce costs.

B) Incorrect. While calling in refills to a doctor helps with patient compliance, it is not the main purpose of MTM.

C) Incorrect. Advising patients of delivery and mail-order options aids compliance, but it is not the purpose of MTM.

D) Correct. MTM is intended to improve patient compliance.

84.
A) Incorrect. Orphan drugs do not necessarily cure diseases; they only treat certain ones.

B) Incorrect. Orphan drugs are rarely used and are not intended for common diseases or conditions.

C) Correct. Orphan drugs are pharmaceuticals that are developed specifically for rare diseases.

D) Incorrect. Orphans drugs are not appropriate for all patients.

85.
A) Incorrect. 120/80 is considered normal blood pressure.

B) Incorrect. 100/70 is not considered high blood pressure.

C) Correct. A reading over 140/90 is considered high.

D) Incorrect. 110/60 would be low blood pressure.

86.
A) Correct. The physician's name is not required in the compounding log. It is required on the prescription label.

B) Incorrect. The lot number of the medication compounded is needed in order to refer back to the product for recall or other purposes as necessary.

C) Incorrect. The pharmacist initials the compound to show that he or she verified it.

D) Incorrect. The beyond-use date is required because once the medication is compounded, the expiration date is different from the date on the manufacturer's packaging.

87. A)   Incorrect. Benztropine does not treat Alzheimer's disease.

    B)   **Correct.** Benztropine is an anti-tremor medication.

    C)   Incorrect. Benztropine is not an anti-anxiety medicine.

    D)   Incorrect. Benztropine is not an anti-depressant.

88. A)   Incorrect. Allergy information is always included in the patient's profile.

    B)   **Correct.** Spousal information is not required for a patient profile.

    C)   Incorrect. The patient's date of birth is required on a patient's profile.

    D)   Incorrect. It is essential that a patient's insurance information be correctly entered on his or her profile.

89. **A)**   **Correct.** It is not realistic to avoid stocking SALAD drugs in the pharmacy.

    B)   Incorrect. Using Tallman lettering is one strategy to differentiate SALAD drugs from other drugs in the pharmacy.

    C)   Incorrect. Color-coding is a strategy to differentiate SALAD drugs from other drugs in the pharmacy.

    D)   Incorrect. Stocking SALAD drugs in a different area in the pharmacy away from the regular stock is one way to differentiate them from other drugs.

90. **C)**

Set up a proportion with mL on top and teaspoons on bottom. Recall that 5 mL = 1 teaspoon.

$$\frac{5 \text{ mL}}{1 \text{ teaspoon}} = \frac{x \text{ mL}}{2 \text{ teaspoons}}$$

Cross-multiply and solve for x.

$x =$ **10 mL**

Note: This can also be solved using Dimensional Analysis, multiplying by conversion ratios to cancel out units until finding the needed units:

$$2 \text{ teaspoons} \times \frac{5 \text{ mL}}{1 \text{ teaspoon}} = 10 \text{ mL}$$

TWO: Practice Test Two

READ THE QUESTION CAREFULLY AND CHOOSE THE MOST CORRECT ANSWER.

1. How would the instructions, "Take 2 tablets in the morning and 1 tablet in the evening as needed" be written using sig codes?

    A) Take 2 tsp qd and 1 tsp qod prn

    B) Take 2 tbsp qam and 1 tbsp qpm prn

    C) Take 2 ts qam and 1 t qpm prn

    D) Take 2 cs qam and 1 c qpm prn

2. In which check system would the technician double check the hard copy against the prescription label generated by the order entry technician?

    A) point-of-sale

    B) verification process

    C) dispensing process

    D) order entry

3. How would 5% be presented in decimals?

    A) 0.005

    B) 0.05

    C) 0.5

    D) 5.0

4. Which of the following is NOT a way for patients to request refills?

    A) The patient may call in an order number on the automated phone system.

    B) The patient may enter the order number information on the pharmacy website.

    C) They patient may give the technician his or her phone number; no other information is needed.

    D) The patient may take a picture of the order number on his or her smart phone and text it to the pharmacy.

5. Which of the following is NOT a characteristic of personal health information (PHI)?

    A) PHI relates to the physical or mental health or condition of an individual.

    B) PHI identifies the individual.

    C) PHI relates to the past, present, and future payments of the individual.

    D) PHI relates to the individual's debit card PIN number.

6. Under which of the following circumstances may pharmacy technicians transfer a refill from a different pharmacy?

A) The refill is from a pharmacy other than the one they work for.

B) The refill is from the same chain pharmacy they work for, it is not a controlled substance, and the computer system is connected.

C) The refill is a controlled substance filled by the same pharmacy chain but at a different store.

D) The refill is a controlled substance originally filled at another pharmacy.

7. Which is used for weighing non-sterile compound ingredients?

A) counter balance

B) compounding slab

C) suppository mold

D) mortar and pestle

8. How many credit hours of continuing education on the topic of medication safety does the PTCB require to be recertified every 2 years?

A) 2

B) 3

C) 4

D) 1

9. Which drug typically contains an agent that resembles the disease that is being treated and causes the pathogen responsible for the disease to weaken or become destroyed in the human body?

A) immunosuppressants

B) antibiotics

C) vaccinations

D) antispasmodics

10. Divide $\frac{2}{15}$ by $\frac{1}{6}$. What is the answer?

A) $\frac{13}{15}$

B) $\frac{1}{2}$

C) $\frac{4}{5}$

D) $\frac{3}{5}$

11. Radiopharmaceuticals are a class of drugs used to treat which of the following?

A) cancer

B) arthritis

C) arrhythmia

D) gastritis

12. Which is NOT an appropriate question to ask a patient who is dropping off a new prescription?

A) Do you have any drug allergies?

B) Has your insurance changed?

C) Are you a drug abuser?

D) Have you had prescriptions filled here before?

13. Which act is an amendment to the Controlled Substance Act?

A) the FDA Modernization Act

B) HIPAA

C) the Combat Methamphetamine Epidemic Act of 2005 (CMEA)

D) the Drug Quality and Security Act

14. Which hormone is NOT released by the hypothalamus?

A) dopamine

B) antidiuretic hormone

C) growth hormone

D) thyrotropin-releasing hormone

15. During which step of the FMEA are actions taken to detect, prevent, or minimize the consequences of any significant errors that may occur during the evaluation?

A) Step 5

B) Step 3

C) Step 1

D) Step 2

16. Which is NOT a law or requirement that was established under the Anabolic Steroids Control Act of 1990?

A) Anabolic steroids are not allowed to be prescribed in the USA.

B) Trainers and advisors cannot recommend anabolic steroid use to individuals.

C) Anabolic steroids must be classified as a CIII controlled substance.

D) Anabolic steroids are defined as a drug or hormonal substance that promotes muscle growth in a way similar to testosterone.

17. A doctor prescribed methylprednisolone 10 mg tables with the following directions:

- 6 tabs po qd for 2 days;
- 5 tabs po qd for 2 days;
- 4 tabs po qd for 2 days;
- 3 tabs po qd for 2 days;
- 2 tabs po qd for 2 days;
- Then 1 tab qd for 5 days

How many tablets should be dispensed to fill this medication?

A) 50

B) 45

C) 100

D) 25

18. How long is a non-controlled prescription valid?

A) two years from the date it is written

B) one year from the date it is written

C) six months from the date it is written

D) thirty days from the date it is written

19. The Physician's Desk Reference (PDR)

A) is a compilation of annually updated manufacturers' prescribing information (package inserts) on prescription drugs.

B) compiles information on 22,000 prescription and 6,000 OTC products. It lists products by therapeutic categories.

C) provides drug information with therapeutic guidelines and off-label uses.

D) gives important dosing information and evaluations for the management of pediatric patients by healthcare professionals.

20. What does the term *osteomalacia* mean?

A) the softening of bone

B) the hardening of bone

C) the breakdown of bone

D) the enlargement of bone

21. Which pharmacy automation helps maintain an accurate accounting of controlled substances and allows the pharmacist to investigate any errors through the pharmacy system?

A) pneumatic tube delivery systems

B) centralized narcotic dispensing and tracking devices

C) web-based compliance and disease management tracking systems

D) electronic clinical documentation systems

22. Which drug does NOT treat osteoporosis?

    A) raloxifene

    B) ibandronate

    C) zoledronic acid

    D) methotrexate

23. What is NOT required to calculate an infusion rate?

    A) volume

    B) strength

    C) flow rate

    D) time

24. Which is NOT considered a HIPAA-covered entity?

    A) healthcare providers

    B) health insurance plans

    C) family members of the patient

    D) healthcare workers

25. Which agency approves the use of investigational new drugs (INDs)?

    A) DEA

    B) CDC

    C) ASPCA

    D) FDA

26. Which reference material gives extensive information on injectable drugs available in the US and internationally?

    A) United States Pharmacists' Pharmacopeia (USP)

    B) Micromedex Healthcare Evidence and Clinical Xpert

    C) Trissel's Handbook on Injectable Drugs

    D) Martindale: The Complete Drug Reference

27. What is the product of 0.42 × 0.56?

    A) 2.352

    B) 23.52

    C) 235.2

    D) 0.2352

28. Which sig code means dispense such doses?

    A) dtd

    B) ATC

    C) LCD

    D) DAW

29. Which of the following is NOT required by the Dietary Supplement Health and Education Act of 1994?

    A) Dietary supplements must be labeled as such, with a statement including the words dietary supplement.

    B) Dietary supplements require a prescription.

    C) Dietary supplements must include a complete list of ingredients by their common names in order of prominence or with the dietary ingredient source in Supplement Facts.

    D) Dietary supplements must include this disclaimer on the label: "This statement has not been evaluated by the FDA. This product is not intended to diagnose, treat, cure or prevent any disease."

30. Which is NOT required to be on a medication order label?

    A) the patient's insurance information

    B) the patient's medical account number

    C) the patient's name

    D) the patient's room number

31. What is done in Phase 3 of a clinical trial?

    A) safety studies during sales; ongoing studies after drug is on the market to establish risks, benefits, and best uses

    B) final confirmation of safety and efficacy; test a larger group of 1,000 to 3,000 to confirm safety, effectiveness, and side effects

    C) safety screening; test a small group to evaluate drug dosage safety and identify side effects

    D) establishing efficacy of the drug against a placebo for safety and effectiveness

32. Which is NOT an OSHA safety guideline that pharmacy technicians must follow?

    A) If exposed skin comes into contact with body fluids, scrub with soap and water as soon as possible.

    B) Do not recap, bend, or break contaminated needles or other sharps.

    C) Use mouth pipetting or suck blood or other harmful chemicals from tubing.

    D) Decontaminate contaminated materials before reprocessing or place in biohazard bags and dispose of according to policies and procedures.

33. A pharmacy tech is asked to prepare 3 L of a 30% solution. The active ingredient needed is stored in 8 ounce bottles of the 70% strength solution. How many bottles of the 70% solution will be needed to complete the order?

    A) 10 bottles

    B) 3 bottles

    C) 6 bottles

    D) 12 bottles

34. What is a decentralized pharmacy?

    A) a system that alerts the nurse as to when the medication needs to be administered

    B) the center of pharmacy operations in a hospital or healthcare facility

    C) nursing unit med rooms that contain an automated dispensing machine

    D) the sterile room

35. Which of the following is NOT a right of the patient under HIPAA?

    A) The patient may obtain a copy of his or her health records.

    B) The patient may not receive a report stating why his or her information was shared.

    C) The patient has the right to give or withhold permission before health information is used.

    D) The patient has the right to receive a notice stating how his or her health information may be used and shared.

36. Which is NOT a place that can compound medication?

    A) home healthcare settings

    B) sports medicine clinics

    C) cancer centers

    D) veterinary clinics

37. Which drug is NOT an opioid pain medicine?

    A) hydrocodone

    B) methadone

    C) morphine

    D) tizanidine

38. Which of the following is NOT a reason that automated dispensing machines are used in institutional pharmacy?

   A) for convenience

   B) for inventory purposes

   C) to reduce the chance of giving the wrong drug

   D) to make IV admixtures

39. Which of the following statements about addressing medication errors is NOT true?

   A) It is important to focus on what caused the error and how to improve the work habits that contributed to the problem.

   B) Using systemic reviews to indicate common factors that lead to errors, pharmacies can develop and implement strategies that improve the quality of the pharmacy workflow while helping to prevent the errors from reoccurring.

   C) Methodologies such as FMEA and Root Cause Analysis (RCA) do not help to improve quality or reduce errors in the pharmacy.

   D) Continuous quality improvements (CQI) which allow the pros and cons of current systems to be acknowledged should be discussed among coworkers, and improvements should be implemented.

40. Which is NOT a characteristic to check for when determining if a controlled substance prescription has been forged?

   A) different pen colors

   B) incorrect DEA number

   C) incorrect doctor's handwriting

   D) A prescription for a controlled substance should never contain refills.

41. When was OSHA established?

   A) 1901

   B) 1970

   C) 1938

   D) 1987

42. Which condition is NOT considered an autoimmune disorder?

   A) multiple sclerosis

   B) lupus

   C) osteoarthritis

   D) vasculitis

43. If a patient feels her or his information was used without permission or not protected, which action may NOT be taken?

   A) The patient can have the healthcare worker terminated with no questions asked.

   B) The patient can file a complaint with her or his health insurer or the US government.

   C) The patient may rescind permission to access PHI at any time.

   D) The patient may authorize or prohibit PHI from being shared.

44. What is a characteristic of a paste?

   A) use of a dry ingredient

   B) oily texture

   C) covered in gelatin

   D) thin texture

45. A 1600 mL IV solution is to be given over a 10-hour period. What is the flow rate in mL per min of the solution?

   A) 2.15 mL/min

   B) 1.87 mL/min

   C) 2.08 mL/min

   D) 2.67 mL/min

46. If two solutions are combined at a ratio of 3:1 to make a compounded solution, how many of each is required to make a 250 mL mixture?

    A) 187.5 mL and 62.5 mL

    B) 150 mL and 100 mL

    C) 200 mL and 50 mL

    D) 175 mL and 75 mL

47. Which information is NOT required on a medication order?

    A) route of administration

    B) drug dosage

    C) patient's phone number

    D) patient's weight

48. Pharmacy technicians generally research all of the following EXCEPT

    A) adverse warnings and effects.

    B) interactions.

    C) dissertations.

    D) indications.

49. All of the following are layers of the heart EXCEPT the

    A) epicardium.

    B) exocardium.

    C) pericardium.

    D) endocardium.

50. Which HIPAA penalty tier states that the covered entity acted with willful neglect and corrected the problem within 30 days?

    A) Tier 1

    B) Tier 2

    C) Tier 3

    D) Tier 4

51. The sig code rep, rept means which of the following?

    A) no refill

    B) label

    C) as needed

    D) repeat

52. What is on a patient's compounding label?

    A) physician's DEA number

    B) patient's social security number

    C) patient's allergies

    D) quantity

53. The 340B program

    A) is medication billing done by the hospital billing department. It codes and bills all diagnosis-related services provided to the patient during the hospital stay into groups.

    B) reduces costs: drug manufacturers give discounts to hospitals in exchange for the drug being placed on the hospital formulary.

    C) is a large setting with many different units and departments that are devoted to patient care.

    D) includes all the medications the patient is taking, even OTC products.

54. Chemical structure is defined as

    A) the patented name of the drug given to it by its manufacturer.

    B) the structural determination of a drug based on molecules and chemical compounds.

    C) the purpose of the drug in terms of how it is used to treat a particular disease or conditions.

    D) a detailed written study about the drug.

55. Pharmacy technicians should do all of the following when checking expiration dates on bottles EXCEPT

A) give any expired drugs to physicians or clinics for low income patients.

B) mark items that will expire within 60 days.

C) remove expired items from the shelves.

D) destroy or return expired items to the manufacturer for credit.

56. HIV/AIDS antiviral drugs help to do all the following EXCEPT

A) slow the progression of the disease.

B) prevent secondary infections.

C) cure HIV/AIDS.

D) prevent complications of the virus.

57. Which of the following statements about MSDS is NOT true?

A) MSDS serve as an inventory list of all hazardous materials that may be found in the pharmacy setting.

B) MSDS are a part of the Bloodborne Pathogen Standard.

C) MSDS outline the structure of a chemical substance and also document potential hazards of the substance.

D) The labels on the MSDS must list the chemical name, warnings, and name and address of the manufacturer.

58. If 5 capsules of Amoxicillin contain 2500 mg of Amoxicillin, how many capsules are required to fill a prescription for 50,000 mg?

A) 50 capsules

B) 25 capsules

C) 100 capsules

D) 75 capsules

59. Volume of distribution in pharmacokinetics

A) is a highly permeable cell barrier that makes up the walls of brain capillaries.

B) is how drug efficiency is affected by the way the proteins bind within plasma.

C) is the hypothetical amount of volume needed to administer the total supply of a drug at the same absorption rate that is observed in blood plasma.

D) is the inactive transport of a biochemical substance without the need for energy input.

60. The Affordable Care Act was initiated to

A) update the Food, Drug, and Cosmetic Act to include technological, trade and public health issues more relevant to the twenty-first century.

B) give the option of a prescription drug discount card to low-income patients who need assistance with increasing drug costs.

C) increase the quality and affordability of healthcare by helping to lower the costs of public and private insurance and lower the amount of uninsured persons in the United States.

D) outline steps to build an electronic tracking system to identify and trace specific prescription drugs distributed in the United States.

61. What is the most important preventive measure in infection control?

A) vaccinations

B) proper handwashing

C) TB testing

D) physicals

62. What factor does NOT affect sterile compounding?

    A) chemical degradation

    B) using the incorrect balance

    C) miscalculation

    D) photo degradation

63. If a patient is picking up a controlled substance, which of the following is NOT necessary?

    A) to ask the patient for a photo ID

    B) to have the patient sign for the medication

    C) to ask a patient's authorized representative to display the patient's photo ID to pick up the prescription

    D) to ask the patient to show his or her Social Security card

64. How many mL of a solution containing 150 mcg/mL of medication would be needed if a patient requires a dose of 1 mg?

    A) 5 mL

    B) 6.67 mL

    C) 3.33 mL

    D) 7.5 mL

65. Which drug is NOT a diuretic?

    A) spironolactone

    B) furosemide

    C) fosinopril

    D) hydrochlorothiazide

66. One dram is equivalent to how much of an ounce?

    A) one-fourth

    B) one-eighth

    C) one half

    D) three quarters

67. Secondary resources are

    A) indexing services or abstracts of publications that require a subscription.

    B) general resources.

    C) a data compilation of the premarket studies and prescribing information.

    D) publications in their original form including technical reports, theses and dissertations, conference papers, and monographic series.

68. Which agency regulates the practice of pharmacy by state?

    A) the ATF

    B) the DEA

    C) the CMS

    D) the BOP

69. Which is NOT an acceptable example as to why a new prescription may not be ready in time for pick up?

    A) The pharmacist needs to contact the physician.

    B) The pharmacist or technician needs to contact the insurance company.

    C) The pharmacist is too busy to verify the prescription for the patient.

    D) The patient must be contacted to ask a question.

70. Which is NOT a general regulation standard enforced by OSHA that pertains to all workplaces?

    A) fire safety and emergency plans

    B) work-related musculoskeletal injuries

    C) violence in the workplace

    D) sexual harassment in the workplace

71. Which of the following is considered an IV fluid?

   A) Heparin

   B) bacteriostatic water

   C) normal saline

   D) sterile water

72. Which of the following medicines is NOT used topically for fungal infections?

   A) clotrimazole

   B) nystatin

   C) terbinafine

   D) triple antibiotic cream

73. Package inserts

   A) are not a tertiary source.

   B) do not provide pharmacodynamics information about the drug.

   C) do not provide overdose information about the drug.

   D) do give information on premarket studies of the drug.

74. How many grams are required to make 500 mL of a 1:5000 solution?

   A) 10 g

   B) 1 g

   C) 0.1 g

   D) 0.01 g

75. Pharmacy technicians can avoid ethical and legal issues due to healthcare fraud by doing all the following EXCEPT

   A) staying current on new laws.

   B) identifying and double-checking procedures while processing claims.

   C) acting on instinct when unsure in a situation.

   D) obtaining prior authorizations when needed.

76. If 50 Lipitor 10 mg tablets cost $75.00, how much would 30 tablets cost?

   A) $50

   B) $40

   C) $25

   D) $45

77. When verifying a prescription, the pharmacist does all of the following EXCEPT

   A) return the stock bottle to the shelf.

   B) compare the hard copy to the label.

   C) check the NDC number on the stock bottle with the NDC number on the label.

   D) check the patient's profile for drug utilization reviews (DURs).

78. Which is NOT a level one risk in sterile compounding facilities?

   A) bulk compounding

   B) garbing up

   C) using a laminar airflow workbench

   D) media-fill testing

79. The National Association of Boards of Pharmacy (NABP) works with which agency to develop and implement uniform standards relating to pharmacy?

   A) the FDA

   B) the BOP

   C) the DEA

   D) the CMS

80. Define *tympanoplasty* by defining the root word and suffix.

   A) puncturing of the ear drum

   B) surgical repair of the jaw

   C) surgical repair of the ear drum

   D) puncturing of the jaw

81. Which of the following is NOT required on a prescription label?

    A) patient's name
    B) directions for use
    C) insurance information
    D) patient's order number

82. The prefix *para–* means which of the following?

    A) to go forth
    B) near, beside
    C) behind, backward
    D) many, excessive

83. If you are compounding a batch of drug A with 280 g and it costs $112.00 per lb., how much will the batch of drug A cost?

    A) $69.14
    B) $47.52
    C) $62.75
    D) $56.88

84. NDC numbers include all of the following information EXCEPT

    A) the labeler number.
    B) the product number.
    C) the package size number.
    D) the pharmacy number.

85. Prescribing authority was established by

    A) the Durham-Humphrey Amendment of 1951.
    B) the Kefauver-Harris Amendment of 1962.
    C) the Affordable Care Act.
    D) the Controlled Substances Act.

86. Which organization is in charge of regulating safety in the workplace?

    A) FDA
    B) CDC
    C) OSHA
    D) DEA

87. A red blood cell is also called

    A) a leukocyte.
    B) a lymphocyte.
    C) an erythrocyte.
    D) a thrombocyte.

88. All of these are chemical materials that are located in the pharmacy EXCEPT

    A) mineral oil
    B) alcohol
    C) gases
    D) radiopharmaceuticals

89. Which is NOT a part of quality assurance in sterile compounding?

    A) proper aseptic technique
    B) education and training
    C) air particulate testing
    D) label generation

90. The drug class suffix *–pam* refers to which of the following?

    A) benzodiazepines
    B) beta blockers
    C) antiviral medications
    D) SSRIs

1.   A)   Incorrect. This would translate to, "Take 2 teaspoonsful every day and 1 teaspoonful every other day as needed."

     B)   Incorrect. This would translate to, "Take 2 tablespoonsful every morning and 1 tablespoonful every night as needed."

     C)   Correct. This would translate to, "Take 2 tablets every morning and 1 tablet every evening as needed."

     D)   Incorrect. This would translate to, "Take 2 capsules every morning and 1 capsule every evening as needed."

2.   A)   Incorrect. At point-of-sale, the technician asks for a second identifier in addition to the patient's name to ensure that the medication was filled for the correct patient.

     B)   Incorrect. In the verification process, the pharmacist checks the prescription order from entry through dispensing.

     C)   Correct. In the dispensing process check system, the technician double checks the hard copy with the prescription label generated by the order entry technician.

     D)   Incorrect. At order entry, the technician uses his or her skill and awareness to ensure the entry of correct information. Furthermore, the label has not yet been generated.

3.   **B)**

     Turn 5% into a decimal by dividing 5 by 100 (per cent means per 100).

     $5\% = \frac{5}{100} = 0.05$

     = 0.05 (B)

4.   A)   Incorrect. Patients can call in a refill request on the automated phone system.

     B)   Incorrect. Patients can enter the order number on the pharmacy website.

     C)   Correct. A patient's phone number is not enough information; a technician will not know which drug to fill.

     D)   Incorrect. Patients can take a picture of the refill bottle with their smart phones and text it to the pharmacy.

5.   A)   Incorrect. One characteristic of PHI is that it does relate to the physical or mental health or condition of an individual.

     B)   Incorrect. PHI does identify the individual.

     C)   Incorrect. PHI relates to the past, present, and future payments of the individual.

     D)   Correct. The PIN number of an individual's debit card is not considered PHI.

6.   A)   Incorrect. Only pharmacists can transfer refills from another pharmacy.

     B)   Correct. Pharmacy technicians can transfer non-control prescriptions from the same pharmacy if the system is connected.

     C)   Incorrect. Only pharmacists can transfer a controlled substance within the same pharmacy chain (if federal and state laws allow).

     D)   Incorrect. Only pharmacists can fill controlled substances from another pharmacy (again, if state and federal laws allow).

7.   A)   Correct. A balance is used for weighing ingredients.

     B)   Incorrect. Compounding slabs are used for combining ingredients.

     C)   Incorrect. A suppository mold is used for making suppositories.

     D)   Incorrect. A mortar and pestle is used for grinding and crushing ingredients.

8.   A)   Incorrect. The PTCB does not require 2 credit hours of continuing education on medication safety for recertification.

     B)   Incorrect. The PTCB does not require 3 credit hours of continuing education on medication safety for recertification.

C) Incorrect. The PTCB does not require 4 credit hours of continuing education on medication safety for recertification.

D) Correct. The PTCB requires 1 credit hour of continuing education on medication safety every 2 years for recertification.

9. **A)** Incorrect. Immunosuppressants treat autoimmune disorders and are used in organ transplants.

B) Incorrect. Antibiotics treat bacterial infections.

C) Correct. Vaccinations typically contain an agent that resembles the disease that is being treated and causes the pathogen responsible for the disease to weaken or become destroyed in the human body.

D) Incorrect. Antispasmodics treat muscle spasms.

10. **C)**

To divide fractions, flip the second fraction and multiply. To multiply, multiply numerators across and denominators across.

$$\frac{2}{15} \div \frac{1}{6} = \frac{2}{15} \times \frac{6}{1} = \frac{12}{15}$$

Reduce (simplify) answer to simplest terms.

$$\frac{12}{15} = \frac{3 \times 4}{3 \times 5} = \frac{4}{5}$$

11. **A) Correct.** Radiopharmaceuticals are used to treat cancer.

B) Incorrect. Radiopharmaceuticals are not used for arthritis.

C) Incorrect. Radiopharmaceuticals do not treat arrhythmia.

D) Incorrect. Radiopharmaceuticals are not used to treat gastritis.

12. **A)** Incorrect. It is important to ask if the patient has drug allergies.

B) Incorrect. Pharmacy technicians should always ask if the patient's insurance has changed.

C) Correct. Pharmacy technicians should never ask patients if they abuse drugs. They should always be extra vigilant when filling controls by checking for forged prescriptions, no matter who the patient is.

D) Incorrect. It is appropriate to ask if a patient has had prescriptions filled at the pharmacy before.

13. **A)** Incorrect. The FDA Modernization Act updated the Food, Drug, and Cosmetic Act to include technological, trade, and public health issues more relevant to the twenty-first century.

B) Incorrect. HIPAA protects patient privacy.

C) Correct. CMEA is an amendment to the Controlled Substance Act.

D) Incorrect. The Drug Quality and Security Act outlined the development of an electronic tracking system that will identify and trace specific prescription drugs distributed in the United States.

14. **A)** Incorrect. Dopamine is produced in the hypothalamus.

B) Correct. Antidiuretic hormone is produced by the pituitary gland.

C) Incorrect. Growth hormone is produced by the hypothalamus.

D) Incorrect. The hypothalamus produces thyrotropin-releasing hormone.

15. **A) Correct.** If any significant errors occur during the evaluation, actions will be taken to detect, prevent, or minimize the consequences during Step 5.

B) Incorrect. During Step 3, the team determines the likelihood and consequences of any mistakes occurring due to failures identified in the process.

C) Incorrect. In Step 1, the team determines how the product is to be used.

D) Incorrect. In Step 2, the team examines possible failures of the drug.

16. **A) Correct.** Anabolic steroids may still be prescribed in the USA.

B) Incorrect. According to the Anabolic Steroids Control Act of 1990, trainers and advisors cannot recommend anabolic steroid use to individuals.

C) Incorrect. Anabolic steroids must now be listed as a CIII controlled substance.

D) Incorrect. The Anabolic Steroids Control Act of 1990 does define anabolic steroids as a drug or hormonal substance that promotes muscle growth in a way similar to testosterone.

17. **B)**

"po" stands for taken by mouth and "qd" stands for once a day (for example, take 6 tablets orally once a day for 2 days).

Compute the number of tablets for each part of the prescription.

Add up the total number of tablets for all the days.

- o 6 tabs po qd for 2 days: 6 × 2 = 12
- o 5 tabs po qd for 2 days: 5 × 2 = 10
- o 4 tabs po qd for 2 days: 4 × 2 = 8
- o 3 tabs po qd for 2 days: 3 × 2 = 6
- o 2 tabs po qd for 2 days: 2 × 2 = 4
- o 1 tab po qd for 5 days: 1 × 5 = 5

45

18. A) Incorrect. Prescriptions expire less than two years from the date they are written.

   B) Correct. Non-controlled prescriptions are good for one year from the date they are written.

   C) Incorrect. Non-controlled prescriptions are valid for longer than six months from the date they are written.

   D) Incorrect. Non-controlled prescriptions may still be filled thirty days after they are written.

19. **A) Correct.** The PDR is a compilation of annually updated manufacturers' prescribing information (package inserts) on prescription drugs.

   B) Incorrect. Drug Facts and Comparisons compiles information on 22,000 prescription and 6,000 OTC products and lists products by therapeutic categories.

   C) Incorrect. American Hospital Formulary Service Drug Information provides drug information with therapeutic guidelines and off-label uses.

D) Incorrect. The Pediatric and Neonatal Dosage Handbook gives important dosing information and evaluations for the management of pediatric patients by healthcare professionals.

20. **A) Correct.** Osteomalacia is the softening of bone.

   B) Incorrect. Osteosclerosis is the hardening of bone.

   C) Incorrect. Osteolysis is the breakdown of bone.

   D) Incorrect. Osteomegaly is the enlargement of bone.

21. A) Incorrect. Pneumatic tube delivery systems help to avoid contamination of products by delivering products in a tube similar to ones used at drive-through pharmacies and banks.

   B) Correct. Centralized narcotic dispensing and tracking devices help ensure accurate counts of controlled substances and provide a mechanism for pharmacists to track errors in inventory.

   C) Incorrect. Web-based compliance and disease management tracking systems help track patient compliance in taking maintenance medications; they also track disease management through software systems connected to physicians' offices, hospitals, and pharmacies.

   D) Incorrect. Electronic clinical documentation systems reduce errors in medication distribution and nurse documentation.

22. A) Incorrect. Raloxifene does treat osteoporosis.

   B) Incorrect. Ibandronate is used to treat osteoporosis.

   C) Incorrect. Zoledronic acid does treat osteoporosis.

   D) Correct. Methotrexate is an immunosuppressant.

23. A) Incorrect. Knowledge of the total volume needed is necessary to calculate the infusion rate.

B) **Correct.** It is not necessary to know the strength of the medication to calculate an infusion rate.

C) Incorrect. The rate at which the fluid drops per minute or hour is required to calculate the infusion rate.

D) Incorrect. It is necessary to know how long the IV will be infused to calculate the infusion rate.

24. A) Incorrect. Healthcare providers are HIPAA-covered entities.

B) Incorrect. Health insurance plans are HIPAA-covered entities.

C) **Correct.** Family members are not HIPAA-covered entities.

D) Incorrect. Healthcare workers are HIPAA-covered entities.

25. A) Incorrect. The DEA (Drug Enforcement Administration) monitors the legal use of controlled substances and prevents their abuse.

B) Incorrect. The CDC (Centers for Disease Control and Prevention) is a government agency that works to protect public health.

C) Incorrect. The ASPCA (American Society for the Prevention of Cruelty to Animals) combats animal abuse and neglect.

D) **Correct.** The FDA (Food and Drug Administration) approves the use of INDs.

26. A) Incorrect. The USP provides information about the standards of strength, purity, and quality of drugs.

B) Incorrect. Micromedex Healthcare Evidence and Clinical Xpert is an online database that includes evidence-based referenced information on drugs, diseases, acute care, toxicology, and alternative medicines for healthcare professionals.

C) **Correct.** Trissel's Handbook on Injectable Drugs gives extensive information on injectable drugs available in the US and internationally.

D) Incorrect. Martindale: The Complete Drug Reference provides information on drugs used internationally.

27. **D)**

Multiply 42 by 56, and then move decimal point 4 places to the left (since .42 has decimal two places to the left and .56 has decimal two places to the left).

$42 \times 56 = 2352.0$

Decimal 4 places to left = **0.2352**

28. **A)** **Correct.** *dtd* means dispense such doses.

B) Incorrect. *ATC* means around the clock.

C) Incorrect. *LCD* means coal tar solution.

D) Incorrect. *DAW* is dispense as written.

29. A) Incorrect. This statement is a requirement of the Dietary Supplement Health and Education Act of 1994.

B) **Correct.** The Dietary Supplement Health and Education Act of 1994 does not require prescriptions for dietary supplements.

C) Incorrect. The Dietary Supplement Health and Education Act of 1994 requires this list.

D) Incorrect. This disclaimer is required by the Dietary Supplement Health and Education Act of 1994.

30. **A)** **Correct.** A patient's insurance information is not required on a medication order label.

B) Incorrect. A patient's medical account number must be included on a medication order label.

C) Incorrect. The patient's name must be visible on a medication order label.

D) Incorrect. A medication order label must include the patient's room number.

31. A) Incorrect. This describes Phase 4 of a clinical trial.

B) **Correct.** This describes Phase 3 of a clinical trial.

C) Incorrect. This describes Phase 1 of a clinical trial.

D) Incorrect. This describes Phase 2 of a clinical trial.

32. A) Incorrect. This is a safety guideline.

B) Incorrect. This is a safety guideline.

C) **Correct.** DO NOT use mouth pipetting or suck blood or other harmful chemicals from tubing.

D) Incorrect. This is a safety guideline.

33. **C)**

Identify the variables.

x = volume of stock solution (it will be necessary to convert to number of 8-ounce bottles after finding the number of liters).

C_1 = concentration of stock solution (active ingredient) = 70%

V_1 = volume of stock solution needed to make new solution = x L

C_2 = final concentration of new solution = 30%

V_2 = final volume of new solution = 3 L

Plug the values into the appropriate formula.

$C_1V_1 = C_2V_2$

$0.7 \times x = 0.30(3)$

Isolate x to get the solution.

$x = \frac{0.9}{0.7} = 1.286$ L

Note that the answer is in liters, and the answer choices are in 8 fluid ounce bottles, so either set up a proportion or use Dimensional Analysis (shown) to get the number of bottles. Recall that there are 33.814 ounces in 1 liter.

Round up to the next bottle.

$1.286 \, \cancel{L} \times \frac{33.814 \text{ ounces}}{1 \, \cancel{L}} \times \frac{1 \text{ bottle}}{8 \text{ ounces}}$

$\approx$ **6 bottles**

34. A) Incorrect. The Medication Administration Record (MAR) alerts the nurse when medication needs to be administered.

B) Incorrect. The central pharmacy is the center of pharmacy operations.

C) **Correct.** The nursing unit med rooms with automated dispensing machines are the decentralized pharmacy.

D) Incorrect. The sterile room is in the central pharmacy.

35. A) Incorrect. Under HIPAA, the patient has the right to obtain a copy of his or her health records.

B) **Correct.** Under HIPAA, the patient does have the right to receive a report stating why his or her information was shared.

C) Incorrect. Under HIPAA, the patient has the right to give or withhold permission before health information is used.

D) Incorrect. Under HIPAA, the patient does have the right to receive a report stating why his or her information was shared.

36. A) Correct. Although CSPs can be infused at a patient's home, they cannot be made there since the home is not an aseptic environment.

B) Incorrect. Sports medicine clinics can prepare compounded medication if they have an aseptic environment.

C) Incorrect. Many cancer centers prepare radiopharmaceuticals on their premises instead of ordering them from compounding pharmacies.

D) Incorrect. Veterinary clinics compound medications and infusions for non-human animals.

37. A) Incorrect. Hydrocodone is an opioid pain medicine.

B) Incorrect. Methadone is an opioid pain medicine.

C) Incorrect. Morphine is an opioid pain medicine.

D) **Correct.** Tizanidine is an antispasmodic.

38. A) Incorrect. Automated dispensing machines are more convenient.

B) Incorrect. Automated dispensing machines help keep track of drugs on units.

C) Incorrect. Automated dispensing machines reduce the chance of medication errors.

D) **Correct.** Automated dispensing machines do not make IV admixtures.

39. A) Incorrect. If an error occurs, determining its cause and how to improve the work habits that contributed to the problem is crucial.

B) Incorrect. Systematic reviews help pharmacies develop and implement strategies to improve pharmacy workflow and prevent the errors from reoccurring.

C) Correct. Methodologies such as FMEA and Root Cause Analysis (RCA) can indeed help improve quality and reduce errors in the pharmacy.

D) Incorrect. Continuous quality improvements (CQI) should be noted and implemented.

40. A) Incorrect. Different pen colors could signify a forged prescription.

B) Incorrect. If the DEA number is incorrect, it could be a forged prescription.

C) Incorrect. If the doctor's handwriting and signature seem wrong, the prescription could be forged.

D) Correct. Some classes of narcotics can have up to six months of refills.

41. A) Incorrect. OSHA was not established in 1901.

B) Correct. OSHA was established in 1970.

C) Incorrect. OSHA was not established in 1938.

D) Incorrect. OSHA was not established in 1987.

42. A) Incorrect. Multiple sclerosis is an autoimmune disorder.

B) Incorrect. Lupus is an autoimmune disorder.

C) Correct. Osteoarthritis is not an autoimmune disorder.

D) Incorrect. Vasculitis is an autoimmune disorder.

43. **A) Correct.** The patient cannot get the healthcare worker terminated with no questions asked.

B) Incorrect. The patient can file a complaint with either of these bodies.

C) Incorrect. The patient can always rescind permission to access PHI.

D) Incorrect. The patient may authorize or prohibit PHI from being shared.

44. **A) Correct.** Pastes are thick, moist, and mixed with a dry ingredient.

B) Incorrect. Ointments have an oily base.

C) Incorrect. Capsules are covered in gelatin.

D) Incorrect. Pastes have a thick texture.

45. **D)**

Identify the formula and variables.

Note that **flow rate** is the volume of the IV solution divided by the time it takes to infuse it.

Since the time is provided in hours, convert it into minutes by multiplying it by 60.

$$\text{flow rate (mL/min.)} = \frac{\text{volume of IV solution}}{\text{time (minutes)}}$$

volume = 1600 mL

time = 10 hours = 600 minutes

Multiply out. Notice that the units turn out correctly!

$$\text{flow rate (mL/min.)} = \frac{1600 \text{ mL}}{600 \text{ min.}} =$$

2.67 mL/min

46. **A)**

Ratio Method:

3:1 means 4 parts total; the first solution has 3 parts, and the second has 1 part.

Set up as proportions with part on top and whole on the bottom. Cross-multiply for each proportion.

$\frac{3}{4} = \frac{x}{250}$; $4x = 750$; $x = $ **187.5 mL**

$\frac{1}{4} = \frac{x}{250}$; $4x = 250$; $x = $ **62.5 mL**

Algebra Method:

Set up equations with a variable that represents how much each solution is "weighted": since the ratio is 3:1, the first is weighted 3 times, and the second is weighted 1 time.

Solve for x and then multiply by 3 and 1, respectively.

$3x + 1x = 250$

$4x = 250$

$x = 62.5$; $3x = $ **187.5 mL**; $1x = $ **62.5mL**

47.
A) Incorrect. A medication order should include the route of administration.

B) Incorrect. Medication orders must include drug dosage information.

C) Correct. The patient's phone number is not required on a medication order.

D) Incorrect. The patient's weight must be included on a medication order.

48.
A) Incorrect. Technicians commonly research adverse effects and warnings.

B) Incorrect. Technicians should regularly study drug interactions.

C) Correct. Technicians do not research dissertations.

D) Incorrect. Technicians regularly research drug indications.

49.
A) Incorrect. The epicardium lies within the pericardium.

B) Correct. The exocardium is not a layer of the heart.

C) Incorrect. The pericardium surrounds the heart.

D) Incorrect. The endocardium lines the inside of the heart.

50.
A) Incorrect. At Tier 1, the entity did not know of the breach.

B) Incorrect. At Tier 2, the entity knew of the breach but did not act with willful neglect.

C) Correct. At Tier 3, the entity acted with willful neglect and corrected the breach within 30 days.

D) Incorrect. At Tier 4, the entity acted with willful neglect and did not correct the breach.

51.
A) Incorrect. The sig code for no refill is NR.

B) Incorrect. The sig code for label is sig.

C) Incorrect. The sig code for as needed is prn.

D) Correct. The sig code for repeat is rep, rept.

52.
A) Incorrect. Controlled substances require the physician's DEA number.

B) Incorrect. Revealing a patient's social security number could be a HIPAA violation.

C) Incorrect. Patient allergy information is stored in the patient's profile.

D) Correct. The quantity of the compounded medication would be on the medication label.

53.
A) Incorrect. This answer choice describes the construction of diagnosis-related groups (DRG).

B) Correct. In the 340B program, drug manufacturers give discounts to hospitals, which place their drugs on the hospital formulary. This program is meant to reduce costs.

C) Incorrect. A health system is a large setting with many different units and departments devoted to patient care.

D) Incorrect. This answer choice describes a medication order.

54.
A) Incorrect. The patented name of the drug given to it by its manufacturer is the drug's brand name.

B) Correct. Chemical structure is the structural determination of a drug based on molecules and chemical compounds.

C) Incorrect. A drug's indication is its purpose or use in treating disease.

D) Incorrect. A detailed written study about the drug is a monograph.

55.
A) Correct. Giving away expired drugs is against the law.

B) Incorrect. The pharmacy technician must mark any items expiring in 60 days.

C) Incorrect. It is the responsibility of the pharmacy technician to pull expired medications from the shelves.

D) Incorrect. Pharmacy technicians must destroy or return expired medications to the manufacturer.

56.

A) Incorrect. HIV/AIDS drugs do help slow the progression of the disease.

B) Incorrect. HIV/AIDS drugs help to prevent secondary infections.

C) Correct. There is no cure for HIV/AIDS.

D) Incorrect. HIV/AIDS drugs can help prevent complications from the virus.

57.

A) Incorrect. MSDS do serve as an inventory list of all hazardous materials that may be found in the pharmacy setting.

B) Correct. MSDS are not part of the Bloodborne Pathogen Standard.

C) Incorrect. MSDS outline the structure of a chemical substance and also document potential hazards of the substance.

D) Incorrect. MSDS labels must list the chemical name, warnings, and name and address of the manufacturer.

58. C)

Set up a proportion with the number of capsules on top and mg on the bottom. We are told that 5 capsules of Amoxicillin contains 2500 mg of Amoxicillin.

$$\frac{5 \text{ capsules}}{2500 \text{ mg}} = \frac{x \text{ capsules}}{50,000 \text{ mg}}$$

Cross-multiply and solve for x.

$2500x = 250,000$

$x = \mathbf{100\ capsules}$

Note: This can also be solved using Dimensional Analysis, multiplying by conversion ratios to cancel out units until finding the needed units:

$\frac{5 \text{ capsules}}{2500 \text{ mg}} \times 50,000 \text{ mg} = 100 \text{ capsules}$

59.

A) Incorrect. The highly permeable cell barrier that makes up the walls of brain capillaries is called the blood-brain barrier.

B) Incorrect. Plasma protein binding describes how drug efficiency is affected by the way the proteins bind within plasma.

C) Correct. Volume of distribution is the hypothetical amount of volume needed to administer the total supply of a drug at the same absorption rate that is observed in blood plasma.

D) Incorrect. Passive diffusion is the inactive transport of a biochemical substance without the need for energy input.

60.

A) Incorrect. The FDA Modernization Act of 1997 updated the Food, Drug, and Cosmetic Act to include technological, trade, and public health issues more relevant to the twenty-first century.

B) Incorrect. The Medicare Modernization Act gave the option of a prescription drug discount card to low-income patients who need assistance with increasing drug costs.

C) Correct. The Affordable Care Act increased the quality and affordability of healthcare by helping to lower the costs of public and private insurance and lower the amount of uninsured persons in the United States.

D) Incorrect. The Drug Quality and Security Act of 2013 outlined steps to build an electronic tracking system that will identify and trace specific prescription drugs distributed in the United States.

61.

A) Incorrect. Although vaccinations are a good tool for infection control, they are not considered the most important preventative measure.

B) Correct. The most important line of defense in preventing contamination and controlling infection is proper aseptic handwashing.

C) Incorrect. Although TB testing for hospital workers is a preventative measure to control the spread of tuberculosis, handwashing is still the most important measure for contamination prevention and infection control.

D) Incorrect. Physicals are personal preventative healthcare measures, but they are not required for infection control.

62.

A) Incorrect. Chemical degradation such as crystallization, clouding, aging, and expiration, etc. can cause instability and contamination of the CSP.

B) Correct. A balance weighs medication in a non-sterile compounding environment, so it would not affect a sterile compound.

C) Incorrect. Miscalculation of an ingredient in a sterile compound can cause severe reactions and possibly death. That is why it is so important to have checkpoints in the pharmacy to prevent such errors.

D) Incorrect. Medications that are sensitive to light can lose potency if not protected.

63.
A) Incorrect. The patient must show a photo ID to receive controlled medications.

B) Incorrect. The patient must sign for a controlled medication.

C) Incorrect. If the patient has authorized another person to pick up his or her prescription, the representative must also present the patient's photo ID.

D) Correct. Patients do not need to show their Social Security cards to pick up controlled substances.

64.
B)

Set up a proportion with mg (weight) on top and mL (volume) on the bottom.

We need to convert 150 mcg to 0.150 mg so units will match.

150 mcg = 0.150 mg

$$\frac{0.15 \text{ mg}}{1 \text{ mL}} = \frac{1 \text{ mg}}{x \text{ mL}}$$

Cross-multiply and solve for *x*.

$0.15x = 1$ mg

x = **6.67 mL**

Note: This can also be solved using Dimensional Analysis, multiplying by conversion ratios to cancel out units until finding the needed units:

$$\frac{1 \text{ mL}}{150 \text{ mcg}} \times \frac{1000 \text{ mcg}}{1 \text{ mg}} \times 1 \text{ mg} = 6.67 \text{ mL}$$

65.
A) Incorrect. Spironolactone is a diuretic.

B) Incorrect. Furosemide is a diuretic.

C) Correct. Fosinopril is an ACE inhibitor.

D) Incorrect. Hydrochlorothiazide is a diuretic.

66.
A) Incorrect. One-fourth of an ounce is not equivalent to one dram.

B) Correct. One dram equals one-eighth of an ounce.

C) Incorrect. One half of an ounce is more than one dram.

D) Incorrect. Three quarters of an ounce is more than one dram.

67.
A) Correct. Secondary resources are indexing services or abstracts of publications that require a subscription.

B) Incorrect. General resources are tertiary resources.

C) Incorrect. Package inserts include a data compilation of premarket studies and prescribing information about a drug.

D) Incorrect. Primary resources are publications in their original form including technical reports, theses and dissertations, conference papers, and monographic series.

68.
A) Incorrect. The ATF does not regulate the state practice of pharmacy.

B) Incorrect. The DEA does not regulate the practice of pharmacy by state.

C) Incorrect. CMS does not regulate the practice of pharmacy by state.

D) Correct. The BOP regulates the practice of pharmacy by state.

69.
A) Incorrect. If there is an issue with the prescription, the pharmacist may have to contact the physician, which could reasonably delay filling the prescription.

B) Incorrect. If the insurance rejects the claim, the prescription may not be ready at the expected time.

C) Correct. If the pharmacy workflow is operating correctly and there are no problems with the prescription, the prescription should be due at the expected time—otherwise, that shows poor customer service.

D) Incorrect. If it is not possible to contact the patient by phone, a reasonable delay in filling the prescription may be expected if the pharmacist needs to speak to the patient.

70. A) Incorrect. General OSHA regulation standards include fire safety and emergency plans.

    B) Incorrect. OSHA regulates work-related musculoskeletal injuries.

    C) Incorrect. General OSHA regulation standards include those that pertain to violence in the workplace.

    D) Correct. General OSHA regulation standards do not address sexual harassment.

71. A) Incorrect. Heparin is an additive that aids blood clotting.

    B) Incorrect. Bacteriostatic water is used for diluting and dissolving medications.

    C) Correct. Normal saline (NS) is one of the most common IV fluids used for CSPs.

    D) Incorrect. Sterile water is normally used for irrigation only.

72. A) Incorrect. Clotrimazole is used for fungal infections.

    B) Incorrect. Nystatin cream does treat fungal infections.

    C) Incorrect. Terbanifine is used to treat fungal infections.

    D) Correct. Triple antibiotic cream is used for bacterial infections.

73. A) Incorrect. Package inserts are a tertiary source.

    B) Incorrect. Package inserts do provide pharmacodynamics information.

    C) Incorrect. Package inserts do provide overdose information.

    D) Correct. Package inserts do give information on premarket studies of the drug.

74. **C)**

    For ratio strengths, remember that the solution is always the larger part, and the drug (active ingredient) is always the smaller (the "1" in the ratio).

Set up a proportion with grams (weight of active ingredient) on top and mL (volume of solution) on the bottom.

$$\frac{1 \text{ gram}}{5000 \text{ mL}} = \frac{x \text{ grams}}{500 \text{ mL}}$$

Cross-multiply and solve for x.

$5000x = 500$

$x = \textbf{0.1 g}$

75. A) Incorrect. Staying current on new laws will ensure compliance with regulations on controlled substances.

    B) Incorrect. Identifying and double-checking procedures will prevent problems.

    C) Correct. Always ask a supervisor if unsure about issues related to controlled substances.

    D) Incorrect. Pharmacy technicians should obtain prior authorizations to avoid problems with controlled substances.

76. **D)**

    Set up a proportion with tablets on top and cost on the bottom. We are told that 50 tablets of Lipitor cost $75 and want to know how much 30 tablets cost.

$$\frac{50 \text{ tablets}}{\$75} = \frac{30 \text{ tablets}}{\$ x}$$

Cross-multiply and solve for x.

$50x = 2250$

$x = \textbf{\$45}$

77. **A) Correct.** The pharmacist is not required to return the stock bottle. The technician normally does.

    B) Incorrect. The pharmacist verifies the hard copy, comparing it with the bottle label.

    C) Incorrect. The pharmacist checks the NDC number on the bottle against the label.

    D) Incorrect. The pharmacist checks DURs on the patient's profile.

78. **A) Correct.** Bulk compounding is considered to be a level two risk.

    B) Incorrect. Pharmacy technicians must garb up for all risk levels.

C) Incorrect. Pharmacy technicians must use a laminar airflow workbench at all risk levels.

D) Incorrect. Media-fill testing is required for all risk levels.

79. A) Incorrect. The NABP does not work with the FDA for this purpose.

B) Correct. The NABP does work with the BOP to develop and implement uniform standards relating to pharmacy.

C) Incorrect. The NABP does not work with the DEA for this purpose.

D) Incorrect. The NABP does not work with CMS for this purpose.

80. A) Incorrect. Tympanoplasty does not mean puncturing of the ear drum.

B) Incorrect. Tympanoplasty does not mean surgical repair of the jaw.

C) Correct. Tympanoplasty means surgical repair of the ear drum.

D) Incorrect. Tympanoplasty does not mean puncturing of the jaw.

81. A) Incorrect. The prescription label must contain the patient's name.

B) Incorrect. The prescription label must indicate directions for use.

C) Correct. It is not necessary to include insurance information on the prescription label.

D) Incorrect. The patient's order number must be on the prescription label.

82. A) Incorrect. The prefix *pro–* means to go forth; it implies progression.

B) Correct. *Para–* means near or beside.

C) Incorrect. The prefix *retro–* means behind or backward.

D) Incorrect. The prefix *poly–* means many or excessive.

83. **A)**

First convert grams into pounds (lbs.) since the cost per lb. is provided. Recall that 1 pound equals 453.592 grams.

Given 280 grams, convert to determine the equivalent pounds.

Set up a proportion with grams on top and pounds on the bottom.

$$\frac{453.592 \text{ grams}}{1 \text{ pound}} = \frac{280 \text{ grams}}{x \text{ pounds}}$$

Cross-multiply and solve for x.

With 0.617 pounds of drug A that costs \$112/lb., the batch of drug A will cost \$0.617 times \$112 = \$69.14.

$453.592x = 280$

$x = 0.617$ pounds

$0.617 \times \$112 = \textbf{\$69.14}$

Note: This can also be solved using Dimensional Analysis, multiplying by conversion ratios to cancel out units until finding the needed units:

$$\frac{\$112}{1 \text{ pound}} \times \frac{1 \text{ pound}}{453.592 \text{ grams}} \times 280 \text{ grams} = \$69.14$$

84. A) Incorrect. The NDC number does include the labeler number.

B) Incorrect. The NDC number includes the product number.

C) Incorrect. The NDC number has the package size number.

D) Correct. The NDC number does not include the pharmacy number.

85. **A) Correct.** Prescribing authority was established by the Durham-Humphrey Amendment of 1951.

B) Incorrect. Prescribing authority was not established by the Kefauver-Harris Amendment of 1962.

C) Incorrect. The Affordable Care Act did not establish prescribing authority.

D) Incorrect. The Controlled Substances Act did not establish prescribing authority.

86. A) Incorrect. The FDA regulates medications, dietary supplements, medical devices, and more.

B) Incorrect. The CDC promotes public health.

C) Correct. OSHA regulates safety in the workplace.

D) Incorrect. The DEA enforces the Controlled Substances Act and combats the illicit use of controlled substances.

87. A) Incorrect. A leukocyte is a white blood cell.

B) Incorrect. A lymphocyte is a lymphatic cell.

C) Correct. An erythrocyte is a red blood cell.

D) Incorrect. A thrombocyte is a platelet used for blood clotting.

88. **A) Correct.** Mineral oil is not a chemical material.

B) Incorrect. Alcohol is a chemical material located in the pharmacy.

C) Incorrect. Gases are chemical materials.

D) Incorrect. Radiopharmaceuticals are chemical materials.

89. A) Incorrect. Aseptic technique is very important in quality assurance. It ensures a sterile, quality product.

B) Incorrect. Education and training help keep personnel up to date on new or revised policies and procedures.

C) Incorrect. Air particulate testing helps keep the sterile environment free of contamination.

D) Correct. Label generation is used for preparing CSPs, not for ensuring their quality.

90. **A) Correct.** The drug class suffix –*pam* refers to benzodiazepines.

B) Incorrect. The suffix –*olol* refers to beta blockers.

C) Incorrect. The suffix –*vir* describes antiviral drugs.

D) Incorrect. The suffix –*tine* describes SSRIs.

THREE: Practice Test Three

READ THE QUESTION CAREFULLY AND CHOOSE THE MOST CORRECT ANSWER, OR WORK THE
PROBLEM.

1. Pharmacology is the study of a combination of all these aspects of a drug EXCEPT its

   A) origin.

   B) effects.

   C) uses.

   D) cost.

2. On a hard copy prescription, a prescriber has written *"lorazepam 1mg, take 1 tablet by mouth at bedtime, #30"* for the patient. Which would be the dose?

   A) by mouth

   B) #30

   C) 1 mg

   D) tablet

3. Which is NOT a circumstance that may require non-sterile compounding?

   A) when a product is commercially unavailable

   B) product flavoring

   C) if a different dosage form is needed

   D) if a medication has been recalled

4. Which is NOT considered a drug action?

   A) cellular membrane distribution

   B) antagonizing action

   C) substance replacement

   D) direct harmful chemical reaction

5. Which amendment required the phrase *Caution: Federal Law Prohibits Dispensing without a Prescription* to be placed on all prescription labels?

   A) the Kefauver-Harris Amendment of 1962

   B) the Orphan Drug Act of 1983

   C) the Durham-Humphrey Amendment of 1951

   D) the Pure Food and Drug Act of 1906

6. Which of the following is NOT a cause of medication errors?

   A) a patient's physiological makeup

   B) the end of a medication's course of therapy

   C) calculation errors

   D) social causes

7. Which is considered an undesired effect of a drug?

    A) a chemical reaction

    B) cell mutation

    C) plasma concentration

    D) an interaction with enzymes

8. A therapeutic window is

    A) how long a drug will be effective.

    B) multiple actions occurring at the same time.

    C) a desired drug action.

    D) a quantity of medication that is both an effective dose and an amount that avoids adverse side effects.

9. Which of the following is NOT an important reason to get the correct phone number from the patient when he or she drops off a prescription?

    A) to verify the patient's name in the computer system

    B) to be able to reach the patient in case of questions

    C) to sell the patient new OTC products available at the pharmacy store

    D) to let the patient know when a prescription is ready to be picked up

10. What is 5 grains equivalent to?

    A) 600 – 650 mg

    B) 300 – 325 mg

    C) 225 – 250 mg

    D) 60 – 65 mg

11. Bioavailability relies on all these factors EXCEPT

    A) chemical form.

    B) stability.

    C) liberation.

    D) metabolism.

12. The Poison Prevention Packaging Act of 1970 required

    A) the manufacturing of generic drugs by drug companies and formed the modern system of regulation of generic drugs in the United States.

    B) that manufacturers and pharmacies must place all medication in containers with childproof caps or packaging.

    C) a prescription to purchase opium; it allowed investigation and required consent to study subjects that use or distribute narcotics.

    D) a ban on false claims, package inserts with directions to be included with products, and exact labeling on the product.

13. A wrong dosage form error happens when

    A) the drug was not prepared as prescribed by the physician.

    B) the patient is not correctly complying with drug therapy.

    C) the prescribed route of administration of the drug is incorrect.

    D) the prescribed dose is not administered as ordered.

14. Which is NOT considered a compounding facility?

    A) sports medicine centers

    B) veterinary clinics

    C) physical therapy centers

    D) cancer centers

15. What is 6 drams equivalent to?

    A) 2 ounces

    B) 4 ounces

    C) 1 ounce

    D) $\frac{1}{2}$ ounce

16. For how long is a non-controlled medication prescription viable after it is written by the physician?

    A) a year from the date it is written

    B) six months from the date it is written

    C) until it runs out of refills

    D) A non-controlled medication prescription is only good for one month after it has been written.

17. What percentage of medication errors occur due to prescription errors?

    A) 5 percent

    B) 2 percent

    C) 10 percent

    D) 20 percent

18. Which is a NOT a route of administration?

    A) absorption

    B) intravenous

    C) transdermal

    D) subcutaneous

19. The State Boards of Pharmacy

    A) protect human health and the environment.

    B) enhance patient safety and quality of care in institutional environments.

    C) promote Medicare, Medicaid, and government plans in regards to healthcare coverage.

    D) focus on the public's health and the implementation and enforcement of state laws of the pharmacy practice.

20. Which is NOT a mechanism of pharmacokinetics?

    A) bioequivalence

    B) liberation

    C) excretion

    D) absorption

21. Which of these drugs is NOT a high-alert medication?

    A) neuromuscular blocking agents

    B) heparin

    C) insulin

    D) penicillin

22. Which is NOT considered a SALAD drug?

    A) metformin

    B) clonidine

    C) amoxicillin

    D) hydromorphone

23. Why is it important to have the correct physician location entered on the prescription if the physician has multiple offices?

    A) This information is required by law.

    B) The patient may call the pharmacy to ask for the physician's phone number.

    C) The pharmacy may need to call the physician for refills or questions. Calling the wrong office is inconvenient and wastes time.

    D) The pharmacy must let the doctor know when the patient's prescription is filled.

24. One-half grain is equal to what?

    A) 65 mg

    B) 25 mg

    C) 35 mg

    D) 32.5 mg

25. Which of the following is NOT considered personal protection equipment (PPE)?

    A) bouffant caps

    B) tennis shoes

    C) goggles

    D) masks

26. When processing a controlled medication prescription, which of the following should NOT influence the pharmacy technician when checking to see if the prescription is possibly forged?

    A) if the quantity or refills look altered

    B) if the physician's handwriting and signature look correct

    C) if the prescription looks copied

    D) if the patient is acting nervous

27. Which is NOT an example of a clinical trial?

    A) treatment

    B) prevention

    C) diagnostic

    D) identification

28. Which of the following is NOT true of the Affordable Care Act?

    A) People must purchase healthcare coverage from the government.

    B) Insurers are prohibited from imposing lifetime limits on benefits such as hospital stays.

    C) Insurance plans must cover medical screenings and preventative care.

    D) Dependents can remain on their parent's health insurance plan until their twenty-sixth birthday.

29. Which is NOT a contributing factor to misreading SALAD drugs?

    A) similar packaging

    B) Tallman lettering

    C) bad lighting

    D) placing product on the shelf incorrectly

30. Simplify the fraction $\frac{121}{77}$.

31. In the word *electrocardiogram*, *–gram* is defined as

    A) relating to the heart.

    B) pertaining to.

    C) to record or picture.

    D) the process of viewing.

32. Which is NOT a standard set by USP Chapter 795 for non-sterile compounding?

    A) quality

    B) environmental testing

    C) purity

    D) strength

33. The scope of practice of a practitioner depends on

    A) whether the practitioner can fill prescriptions.

    B) how many prescriptions the practitioner can fill.

    C) whether the practitioner can diagnose or treat a condition.

    D) how long the practitioner has been practicing.

34. If a person has myasthenia, he or she has

    A) motion sickness.

    B) muscle weakness.

    C) a hardening of the arteries.

    D) a stroke.

35. Pharmacy technicians assist pharmacists with all these aspects of MTM EXCEPT which of the following?

    A) compliance

    B) administrative duties

    C) patient counseling

    D) collecting patient data

36. With regard to expiring medications, stock bottles are removed from the shelf

    A) one month before expiring.

    B) two months before expiring.

    C) three months before expiring.

    D) two weeks before expiring.

37. When transferring a prescription from one pharmacy to another, pharmacy technicians can get all the information from the patient and/or patient's prescription bottle for the pharmacist (who then calls for the transfer) EXCEPT for which of the following?

    A) patient's name

    B) amount of refills left on prescription

    C) name of drug

    D) pharmacy name

38. In the word *xerodermatic*, *xer*– would be the

    A) prefix.

    B) suffix.

    C) word root.

    D) combining vowel.

39. Aseptic technique consists of all of the following EXCEPT

    A) good personal hygiene.

    B) a sterile work area.

    C) wearing scrubs.

    D) proper hand washing technique.

40. Which information does NOT need to be checked on a controlled prescription when the patient drops it off?

    A) the manual signature of prescriber

    B) the date the prescription was written

    C) the patient's full name and address

    D) the patient's signature

41. Which of the following describes when a prescription has no refills left and the physician's office gives more refills on the prescription?

    A) a refill request

    B) workflow

    C) a refill authorization

    D) maintenance medications

42. Which of the following is equivalent to 2 ounces?

    A) 30 ml

    B) 60 ml

    C) 120 ml

    D) 240 ml

43. Which stage of FMEA consists of identifying any failures in the process and determining why the failure is occurring?

    A) Stage 1

    B) Stage 4

    C) Stage 3

    D) Stage 2

44. What is the definition of leukocytopenia?

    A) cancer of the white blood cells

    B) bone marrow tumor

    C) excessive white blood cells

    D) decreased number of white blood cells

45. A pharmacy technician incorrectly reads a prescription label. Which multiple-check system has failed?

    A) data entry

    B) verification

    C) drop-off

    D) dispensing

46. The definition of *triturate* is

   A) to grind or crush into a fine paste.

   B) to dissolve one or more chemical liquid substances in water.

   C) to diffuse a liquid into another impassable liquid.

   D) to rub or crush into a fine powder.

47. What is 1.5 quarts equivalent to?

   A) 1440 ml

   B) 960 ml

   C) 1240 ml

   D) 2500 ml

48. What is the first and most important step taken when inputting new prescriptions for patients?

   A) inputting correct prescription information into the correct fields

   B) inputting third-party payer information

   C) adding override codes

   D) being sure to enter the correct information under the correct patient profile

49. When all the word parts are put together to form a word, it is called

   A) a suffix.

   B) a combining form.

   C) word building.

   D) a combining vowel.

50. Which reference material identifies approved drug products and includes evaluations of therapeutic equivalents (generic drugs)?

   A) the *Red Book*

   B) *Ident-A-Drug*

   C) the *Orange Book*

   D) *The Physician's Desk Reference*

51. Current medications are added to a patient's profile for all EXCEPT which of the following reasons?

   A) in case the patient has arthritis and cannot open the bottle

   B) to detect therapeutic duplications

   C) to detect drug duplications

   D) to check for adverse reactions

52. A pharmacy technician negligently filled the wrong strength of a medication and the pharmacist did not catch the mistake while verifying. The patient did not read the paperwork that came along with the prescription and took it anyway; she ended up in the hospital from an overdose and sues the pharmacy.

   Under the respondeat superior doctrine, who or which of the following would NOT be responsible for the mistake?

   A) the pharmacist

   B) the patient

   C) the pharmacy technician

   D) the place of business

53. Which is NOT included in the hazard communication plan?

   A) the location of MSDS

   B) the location of hazard-related information

   C) the location of cleaning equipment

   D) how to fill out a worker's compensation claim

54. Which compound can be made using a mold?

   A) a capsule

   B) a tablet

   C) a solution

   D) a lotion

55. Amniocentesis is

    A)   a water treatment.

    B)   a nerve spasm.

    C)   head pain.

    D)   a surgical procedure for collecting amniotic fluid.

56. Which is NOT a government health plan?

    A)   Medicare

    B)   private employee group health plans

    C)   Medicaid

    D)   TRICARE

57. Simplify the expression: $\frac{2}{3} - \frac{1}{5}$.

58. What is a route of administration for sterile compounding?

    A)   oral

    B)   rectal

    C)   sublingual

    D)   intravenous

59. Which drug is NOT considered a CII drug?

    A)   cocaine

    B)   marijuana

    C)   oxycodone

    D)   hydrocodone

60. Which of the following is NOT among the information most commonly researched by pharmacy technicians?

    A)   monographs

    B)   brand name or generic name of a drug

    C)   drug interactions

    D)   peer reviews by experts

61. Which is NOT one of a pharmacy technician's ethical duties?

    A)   A pharmacy technician never assists in the dispensing, promoting, or distribution of medications or medical devices that are not of good quality or do not meet the standards required by law.

    B)   A pharmacy technician supports and promotes honesty and integrity in the profession, which includes a duty to observe the law, maintain the highest moral and ethical conduct at all times, and uphold the ethical principles of the profession.

    C)   A pharmacy technician associates with and engages in the support of organizations which promote the profession of pharmacy through the utilization and enhancement of pharmacy technicians.

    D)   A pharmacy technician helps the pharmacist by counseling patients to free up time when the pharmacist is backed up verifying prescriptions.

62. In the word *epidermal*, which word part means upon, above?

    A)   *epi–*, the prefix

    B)   *–al*, the suffix

    C)   *derm*, the word root

    D)   all of the above

63. Which must be first verified upon removing the bottle from the shelf when filling a prescription?

    A)   the size of the dram vial

    B)   how many pills to count

    C)   the NDC number

    D)   the patient's name on the label

64. In the word *osteomyelitis*, which word part means muscle?

 A) *osteo*–, the prefix

 B) *myel*, one of the word roots

 C) *–itis*, the suffix

 D) all of the above

65. Which is NOT a methodology used by pharmacies for continuous quality improvement?

 A) root cause analysis

 B) suggestion boxes

 C) FMEA

 D) FOCUS-PDCA

66. Which drug tier is for preferred brand names?

 A) Tier 1

 B) Tier 2

 C) Tier 3

 D) Tier 4

67. All of the following are eligible for Medicaid EXCEPT

 A) patients who are blind.

 B) patients who are disabled.

 C) patients whose incomes are below the poverty level.

 D) patients above the poverty level who do not work.

68. A generic drug must have all the same characteristics as a brand name drug EXCEPT its

 A) active ingredient.

 B) color.

 C) dosage.

 D) strength.

69. Which DEA registrant type is used for a hospital or clinic?

 A) B

 B) M

 C) L

 D) A

70. What quantity is 3 tablespoonsful equivalent to?

 A) 60 ml

 B) 5 ml

 C) 30 ml

 D) 45 ml

71. Which is NOT covered by standard guidelines in USP Chapter 797?

 A) complying with the FDA requirements

 B) air quality

 C) stability and sterilization

 D) proper continuing education

72. When was the USP made a legal standard?

 A) 1901

 B) 1938

 C) 1907

 D) 1975

73. Which is NOT a step to verifying a DEA number using the DEA formula?

 A) Add the second, fourth, and sixth numbers and multiply by 2.

 B) Make sure the second letter of the DEA number is the first letter of the practitioner's last name.

 C) Add the first, third, and fifth numbers together and multiply by 2.

 D) Make sure the first number is a DEA registrant type that is able to prescribe medications to patients.

74. Which type of source is MOST commonly used in research by pharmacy technicians?

    A) tertiary sources

    B) secondary sources

    C) primary sources

    D) none of the above

75. What is a PCN number on the patient's medical ID card?

    A) a number used by PBMs for network benefit routing; it may change depending on what benefit is being billed

    B) a number that directs the claim to the specific insurance benefits for that group (The groups are collections of people who have similar benefits packages such as employee groups.)

    C) a number that directs the claim to the correct third-party provider

    D) a number that indicates the beneficiary who receives the health insurance (This person may not be the patient who brought the prescription in to be filled.)

76. Drugs in a drug class must have all these traits in common EXCEPT

    A) the same targeted mechanism.

    B) a similar mode of action.

    C) the same active ingredient.

    D) similar structures.

77. Which of the following is 24 drams approximately equivalent to?

    A) 2 teaspoonsful

    B) 8 tablespoonsful

    C) 4 tablespoonsful

    D) 8 teaspoonsful

78. Which is NOT a reason for a rejected claim?

    A) refill too soon

    B) quantity limits exceeded

    C) no refills available

    D) prior authorization required

79. The WAC is

    A) based on the selling price data from manufacturers as well as volume discounts and price concessions.

    B) the list price for which the manufacturer sells the drug to the wholesaler.

    C) the average price paid to manufacturers by the wholesalers, which only distribute to retail pharmacies.

    D) the maximum of federal matching funds the federal government will pay to state Medicaid programs for eligible drugs.

80. Find $2\frac{1}{3} - \frac{3}{2}$.

81. Drugs in the class with suffixes *–olone* and *–sone* address all these body systems EXCEPT the

    A) cardiovascular system.

    B) respiratory system.

    C) immune system.

    D) musculoskeletal system.

82. What is a characteristic of bacteria?

    A) It is an infective agent capable of multiplying in the cells of a living host.

    B) It can decompose and absorb organic material as it grows.

    C) It can become a pyrogen if introduced into the bloodstream.

    D) It cannot grow on soft surface areas.

83. A retrospective payment is also known as which of the following?

   A) the point of service

   B) dispensing fee

   C) the APC

   D) fee-for-service

84. Which is NOT considered an example of fraud?

   A) using another person's insurance card

   B) billing a claim with correct information on it

   C) billing for services not rendered

   D) altering monetary amounts on a claim

85. Which drug class suffix does NOT refer to drugs that kill or inhibit the growth of bacterial microorganisms?

   A) –cillin

   B) –vir

   C) –mycin

   D) –cycline

86. 2.5 pints is equivalent to:

   A) 1500 mL

   B) 960 mL

   C) 1200 mL

   D) 480 mL

87. Which is not required to be on a prescription label?

   A) a picture of the drug

   B) the order number

   C) directions for use

   D) the patient's name

88. What is NOT documented on a perpetual inventory log?

   A) CII drug information when ordered from the drug manufacturer

   B) the patient to whom the CII drug was prescribed

   C) CII drugs received by the drug manufacturer

   D) the balance of the quantity for the specific CII drug after each CII drug transaction is recorded

89. Which is NOT a safety guideline required by OSHA for pharmacy technicians?

   A) Technicians may recap, bend, or break contaminated needles or other sharps if necessary.

   B) Technicians must minimize splashing, spraying, or splattering of drops of hazardous chemicals or infectious materials.

   C) Technicians must observe warning labels on biohazard packaging and containers.

   D) Technicians may not keep food or drink in refrigerators, freezers, countertops, shelves, or cabinets that can be exposed to blood, bodily fluid, or hazardous chemicals.

90. Find the sum of $\frac{9}{16}$, $\frac{1}{2}$, and $\frac{7}{4}$.

1.
A) Incorrect. Pharmacology includes the study of a drug's origin—from what it was derived (e.g., a plant, an animal, chemical synthesis).

B) Incorrect. Pharmacology is concerned with the effects of a drug on the body.

C) Incorrect. Pharmacology requires knowledge of a drug's uses.

D) Correct. How much a drug costs is not part of the science of how a drug works in the body.

2.
A) Incorrect. *By mouth* is the route of administration.

B) Incorrect. *#30* indicates the quantity.

C) Incorrect. The dosage strength is 1 mg.

D) Correct. *Tablet* indicates the dose.

3.
A) Incorrect. Compounding is available for specialized compounds such as patient-specific hormonal creams and veterinary products.

B) Incorrect. Flavoring is added to medications to improve taste.

C) Incorrect. If a patient cannot take a tablet, medication can be compounded to make a liquid.

D) Correct. If a medication is recalled, then it may be temporarily unavailable.

4.
A) Correct. Cellular membrane distribution is a desired effect.

B) Incorrect. Antagonizing action is when a drug binds to a receptor without activating it.

C) Incorrect. Substance replacement, or replacing action, refers to a substance's accumulation or storage in the body.

D) Incorrect. Direct harmful chemical reactions, which entail cell destruction, are used with chemotherapy.

5.
A) Incorrect. The Kefauver-Harris Amendment of 1962 gave the FDA the authority to approve a manufacturer's marketing application before the drug was to become available for consumer or commercial use.

B) Incorrect. The Orphan Drug Act of 1983 was passed to help development of treatment for orphan diseases such as Huntington's disease, Tourette's syndrome, muscular dystrophy, and ALS, which only affect a small portion of the population.

C) Correct. The Durham-Humphrey Amendment of 1951 required prescription labels to state Caution: Federal Law Prohibits Dispensing without a Prescription.

D) Incorrect. The Pure Food and Drug Act of 1906 required manufacturers to properly label a drug with truthful information.

6.
A) Incorrect. The patient's physiological makeup can cause a medication error.

B) Correct. The end of a course of medication therapy is not a medication error.

C) Incorrect. Calculation errors may result in medication errors.

D) Incorrect. Medication errors may be due to social causes.

7.
A) Incorrect. A chemical reaction is a desired activity.

B) Correct. Cell mutation is indeed an undesired effect.

C) Incorrect. Plasma concentration is not an effect but is the amount of a drug present in a sample of plasma, and it helps when plotting a drug's duration of action.

D) Incorrect. Interaction with enzymes is also a desired activity.

8.
A) Incorrect. How long a drug is effective is its duration of action.

B) Incorrect. Multiple actions occurring at the same time is considered an undesired effect.

C) Incorrect. A therapeutic window is not a drug action.

D) Correct. A therapeutic window is a workable range calculated by comparing the effective dose of a drug with the amount of it that produces adverse side effects.

9. A) Incorrect. It is important to have a correct phone number for verifying a patient.

    B) Incorrect. It is important to have a number in case a complication arises during the filling process.

    C) Correct. It is not important to call patients on the phone for sales purposes.

    D) Incorrect. It is important to let patients know when their prescriptions are ready.

10. A) Incorrect. This range is too high.

    B) Correct. Five grains is equal to 300 – 325 mg.

    C) Incorrect. This range is too low.

    D) Incorrect. This range is too low.

11. A) Incorrect. Chemical form, even when presented differently as a generic, is a factor of bioavailability.

    B) Incorrect. Stability of a drug is also a factor of bioavailability.

    C) Correct. Liberation—the release of a drug from its pharmaceutical formulation—is a phase of pharmacokinetics but not specific to bioavailability.

    D) Incorrect. Metabolism is another factor of bioavailability.

12. A) Incorrect. The Drug Price Competition and Patent Term Restoration Act of 1984 required the manufacturing of generic drugs by the drug companies and formed the modern system of regulation of generic drugs in the United States.

    B) Correct. The Poison Prevention Packaging Act of 1970 required that manufacturers and pharmacies must place all medication in containers with childproof caps or packaging.

    C) Incorrect. The Harrison Narcotics Tax Act of 1914 required a prescription to purchase opium, allowed investigation

of its legitimacy, taxed it, and required consent to study subjects that use or distribute narcotics.

    D) Incorrect. The Food, Drug, and Cosmetics Act banned false claims, required that package inserts with directions be included with products, and required exact labeling on the product.

13. A) Incorrect. Wrong drug preparation errors happen when the drug was not prepared as prescribed by the physician.

    B) Incorrect. Compliance errors happen when the patient does not correctly comply with drug therapy.

    C) Correct. A wrong dosage form error occurs when the prescribed route of administration of the drug is incorrect.

    D) Incorrect. Omission errors occur when the prescribed dose is not administered as ordered.

14. A) Incorrect. Sports medicine centers compound creams and injections for joint and muscle ailments.

    B) Incorrect. Veterinary clinics compound medications for non-human animals.

    C) Correct. Physical therapy relates to exercises and massages for physical disabilities without the use of medications.

    D) Incorrect. Cancer centers make oncology infusions and injections for cancer patients.

15. A) Incorrect. Two ounces does not equal 6 drams.

    B) Incorrect. Four ounces does not equal 6 drams.

    C) Correct. An ounce does equal 6 drams.

    D) Incorrect. Half an ounce is less than 6 drams.

16. **A) Correct.** A prescription is good for a year after the date it is written.

    B) Incorrect. Certain controlled medication prescriptions are only valid for six months from the date written.

C) Incorrect. Prescriptions may change in strength or be discontinued, so they are only valid for a year.

D) Incorrect. This applies to controlled substances.

17. A) Incorrect. Less than 5 percent of medication errors occur due to prescription errors.

B) **Correct.** Only 2 percent of medication errors are caused by prescription errors.

C) Incorrect. Less than 10 percent of medication errors are caused by prescription errors.

D) Incorrect. Less than 20 percent of medication errors are caused by prescription errors.

18. **A)** **Correct.** Absorption—the process of a drug entering the blood—is a mechanism of pharmacokinetics but not a ROA.

B) Incorrect. An intravenous route is into the vein.

C) Incorrect. A transdermal route is through the skin.

D) Incorrect. A subcutaneous route delivers a drug under the skin.

19. A) Incorrect. The EPA protects human health and the environment.

B) Incorrect. The Joint Commission is a not-for-profit organization; its main function is to enhance patient safety and quality of care in institutional environments.

C) Incorrect. CMS promotes Medicare, Medicaid, and government plans in regards to healthcare coverage.

D) **Correct.** The State Boards of Pharmacy focus on the public's health and the implementation and enforcement of relevant state laws of the pharmacy practice.

20. **A)** **Correct.** When two drugs have the same bioavailability they have the same chemical form and are considered bioequivalent.

B) Incorrect. Liberation is the release of a drug from its pharmaceutical formulation and a mechanism of pharmacokinetics.

C) Incorrect. Excretion is also a mechanism of pharmacokinetics. It is the elimination of a drug from the body.

D) Incorrect. Absorption too is a mechanism of pharmacokinetics and refers to the process of a drug entering the bloodstream.

21. A) Incorrect. Neuromuscular blocking agents are high-alert medications.

B) Incorrect. Heparin is a high-alert medication.

C) Incorrect. Insulin is a high-alert medication.

D) **Correct.** Penicillin is not a high-alert medication.

22. A) Incorrect. Metformin is a SALAD drug.

B) Incorrect. Clonidine is a SALAD drug.

C) **Correct.** Amoxicillin is not a SALAD drug.

D) Incorrect. Hydromorphone is a SALAD drug.

23. A) Incorrect. As long as the correct DR and DEA number are entered, the law does not require the correct location of the physician's office to be on the prescription.

B) Incorrect. It is not the pharmacy's responsibility to give the patient the doctor's number, although for customer service purposes, it is helpful to have it.

C) **Correct.** Calling the wrong office can cause confusion and cost time because the office may not have the patient's records at that location.

D) Incorrect. The doctor does not need to be informed when the patient's prescription is ready.

24. A) Incorrect. Half a grain does not equal 65 mg.

B) Incorrect. Half a grain is not equal to 25 mg.

C) Incorrect. Half a grain is not equal to 35 mg.

D) **Correct.** Half a grain is equivalent to 32.5 mg.

25. A) Incorrect. Bouffant caps are used as PPE. Caps keep hair from contaminating compounded products.

    B) **Correct.** Tennis shoes are not considered PPE.

    C) Incorrect. Goggles are PPE. They protect the eyes from irritants and backsplash.

    D) Incorrect. Masks prevent contamination with bodily fluid and stop the preparer from inhaling irritants.

26. A) Incorrect. Always check to see if anything looks altered on the prescription.

    B) Incorrect. If the handwriting or signature of the physician looks wrong, then question whether the prescription was altered.

    C) Incorrect. If it does not look like the prescription was actually written, then question the prescription. One way to determine this is the absence of indentation from pushing the pen on the paper, or if the writing looks faded.

    D) **Correct.** If a patient has a valid prescription for a controlled medication with no signs of forgery or fraud, a pharmacy cannot turn him or her away just because the patient seems nervous. The patient may feel as though he or she is being discriminated against. If the technician feels uncomfortable filling the prescription, the pharmacist must be notified; he or she will decide whether to fill the prescription. Sometimes, patient behavior could even be a symptom of the disease or condition the doctor is treating. For example, if a patient seems nervous, the medication being filled may be for an anxiety disorder.

27. A) Incorrect. Treatment clinical trials focus on new treatments and/or new combinations of drugs.

    B) Incorrect. Prevention clinical trials deal with ways to prevent diseases.

    C) Incorrect. Diagnostic trials aim to improve on or design new ways of diagnosing conditions.

    D) **Correct.** Identification is one of the details pharmacy technicians must record in the logbook of an investigational drug.

28. **A)** **Correct.** The ACA does not require consumers to buy healthcare coverage from the government.

    B) Incorrect. The ACA does prohibit insurers from imposing lifetime limits on benefits such as hospital stays.

    C) Incorrect. The ACA does require insurance plans to cover medical screenings and preventative care.

    D) Incorrect. The ACA does require that dependents be permitted to remain on the parent's health insurance plan until their twenty-sixth birthday.

29. A) Incorrect. Pharmacy technicians could confuse SALAD drugs because of similar packaging.

    B) **Correct.** Tallman lettering helps differentiate SALAD drugs from each other.

    C) Incorrect. Bad lighting may cause confusion among SALAD drugs.

    D) Incorrect. Placing products on the shelf incorrectly could cause pharmacy technicians to mix up SALAD drugs.

30. $\frac{121}{77} =$

    $\frac{11}{11} \times \frac{11}{7}$

    $= \frac{11}{7}$

    121 and 77 share a common factor of 11. So, if we divide each by 11 we can simplify the fraction.

31. A) Incorrect. The word root *cardi* is related to the heart.

    B) Incorrect. *Pertaining to* relates to the suffixes –*ac*, –*al*, –*ar*, –*ary*, –*eal*, –*ic*, and –*tic*.

    C) **Correct.** The suffix –*gram* means to record or picture.

    D) Incorrect. The suffix –*scopy* translates as a process of viewing.

32. A) Incorrect. USP Chapter 795 requires that the finished product meet a certain level of quality.

B) Correct. Environmental testing is part of USP 797 for air quality in the clean room.

C) Incorrect. USP Chapter 795 requires that the finished product meet a certain level of purity.

D) Incorrect. USP Chapter 795 requires that the finished product be at the appropriate strength.

33. A) Incorrect. Scope of practice is determined by whether the practitioner can diagnose or treat a condition. If the practitioner cannot treat or diagnose a condition, he or she cannot write prescriptions at all.

B) Incorrect. If the practitioner's scope of practice does not allow him or her to write prescriptions, then there would be no prescriptions to fill in the first place.

C) Correct. Scope of practice is determined by whether the practitioner can diagnose or treat a condition.

D) Incorrect. If a practitioner does not treat or diagnose a condition, his or her years of experience are irrelevant.

34. A) Incorrect. None of the common word parts in the tables point to motion sickness in particular, though some refer to abnormality or pain and the word root *gastr* relates to the stomach.

B) Correct. The word root *my* relates to muscles, and the suffix *asthenia* means weakness.

C) Incorrect. Arteriosclerosis is a hardening of the arteries. The suffix –*sclerosis* means hardening, and though *arterio* is not found in these tables, this word part is so similar to the word *artery*, it is easily deciphered.

D) Incorrect. The suffix –*plegia* signifies a stroke or paralysis.

35. A) Incorrect. Pharmacy technicians assist MTM pharmacists with compliance.

B) Incorrect. Pharmacy technicians assist with MTM administrative duties.

C) Correct. Only MTM pharmacists can counsel patients.

D) Incorrect. Pharmacy technicians assist with collecting patient data.

36. **A) Correct.** Expiring medications should be removed from the shelf one month before their expiration date.

B) Incorrect. Expiring medications are not removed from the shelf two months before their expiration date.

C) Incorrect. Expiring medication stock bottles are marked three months before expiration date; they are not yet removed.

D) Incorrect. Expiring medications should have already been removed from the shelf two weeks before their expiration date.

37. A) Incorrect. The technician can take the patient's name.

B) Correct. The pharmacist confirms the amount of refills left when he or she calls the other pharmacy.

C) Incorrect. The technician can get the name of the drug, but the pharmacist will verify when calling the other pharmacy.

D) Incorrect. The technician can ask the patient for the pharmacy name.

38. **A) Correct.** *Xer–* is the prefix, which means dry.

B) Incorrect. The suffix of the word is –*tic*, which means pertaining to.

C) Incorrect. The word root is *derm* or *derma*, which is the Greek word for skin.

D) Incorrect. The combining vowel could be the *a* between *derm–* and –*tic*, but the word root can take the form of either *derm* or *derma*.

39. A) Incorrect. Keeping clean is essential to avoid microbe contamination.

B) Incorrect. A sterile work area keeps the compounded product pure.

C) Correct. Wearing scrubs can still contaminate a sterile environment.

D) Incorrect. Proper handwashing is the best way to avoid contamination.

40. A) Incorrect. The physician should have manually signed the prescription.

B) Incorrect. The original date of the prescription is important because a controlled prescription is only valid for a limited time.

C) Incorrect. The patient's full name and address is required on a controlled prescription.

D) Correct. The patient's signature is not required on a controlled prescription.

41. A) Incorrect. A refill request can either be a patient asking for a refill or the pharmacy calling the physician's office for a refill authorization.

B) Incorrect. Workflow is an organized system in the pharmacy that helps prioritize tasks.

C) Correct. When the physician approves refills for a patient on a prescription that has none left, it is called a refill authorization.

D) Incorrect. Maintenance medications are drugs that the patient needs to take every day for a chronic condition.

42. A) Incorrect. This number is too low.

B) Correct. Two ounces is equivalent to 60 ml.

C) Incorrect. This number is too high.

D) Incorrect. This number is too high.

43. A) Incorrect. In Stage 1 the multidisciplinary team first determines how the product is to be used.

B) Incorrect. Stage 4 is when the team considers the patient's pre-existing conditions, if any, and any processes already in place that may cause an error before the drug reaches the patient.

C) Correct. In Stage 3 the team identifies any failures in the process and determines why those failures are occurring.

D) Incorrect. Stage 2 is when the team examines possible failures of the drug, including whether the drug could be mistaken for another one, if the labeling of the drug could be confused with another, or if errors could easily occur during the administration of the drug.

44. A) Incorrect. *Leuk–* relates to white, but the rest of the word parts do not point to cancer, which is found in the word roots *canc* and *carcin*.

B) Incorrect. The word root *oste* or *osteo* signifies bone, the suffix *–oma* relates to a tumor, and both word parts are missing from leukocytopenia.

C) Incorrect *Leuk–* signifies white, and the word root *cyto* means cell, but the rest of the word does not point to the blood.

D) Correct. The prefix *leuk–* means white, the *o* is a combining vowel, the word root *cyto* means cell, and the suffix *–penia* means a deficiency or decreased number.

45. A) Incorrect. During data entry, pharmacy technicians focus on accurately entering patient data.

B) Incorrect. Pharmacists, not pharmacy technicians, are responsible for verification.

C) Incorrect: Pharmacy technicians work with the patient to accurately enter information during drop-off and alert the pharmacist to any valid concerns.

D) Correct. Pharmacy technicians may incorrectly read the prescription label during the dispensing process when selecting the drug.

46. A) Incorrect. Grinding or crushing into a paste is levigating.

B) Incorrect. Dissolving one or more chemical liquid substances in water results in a solution.

C) Incorrect. Diffusing a liquid into another impassable liquid results in an oil-in-water emulsion.

D) Correct. To rub or crush into a fine powder is to triturate.

47.

$\dfrac{1 \text{ quart}}{960 \text{ mL}} = \dfrac{1.5 \text{ quarts}}{x \text{ mL}}$	Set up a proportion with quarts on top and mL on bottom. Recall that 1 quart = 960 mL.
$x = 1.5 \times 960$ $x = \textbf{1440 mL (A)}$	Cross-multiply and solve for x.

Note: This can also be solved using Dimensional Analysis, multiplying by conversion ratios to cancel out units until finding the needed units. Here, ratios are set up so that unwanted units cross out on top and bottom:

$1.5 \text{ quarts} \times \dfrac{960 \text{ mL}}{1 \text{ quart}} = 1440 \text{ mL}$

48.
A) Incorrect. While accurately inputting prescription information in the correct fields is important, it is not the first or most important step.

B) Incorrect. Although important, inputting third-party payer information in the system is not the most important step, nor is it the first.

C) Incorrect. Pharmacy technicians must be able to code correctly; however, this is not the most important or first step in the process of inputting new prescriptions for patients.

D) **Correct.** The first and most important step in the process is verifying the accuracy of the information under the patient profile.

49.
A) Incorrect. A suffix is the word part found after the root in a word.

B) Incorrect. A combining form is any word element that occurs only in combination with other word elements.

C) **Correct.** Word building is combining all the word parts to form a word.

D) Incorrect. A combining vowel is the vowel used to combine two word parts.

50.
A) Incorrect. The *Red Book* is a resource on drug pricing.

B) Incorrect. *Ident-A-Drug* is a pill identifier.

C) **Correct.** *The Orange Book* identifies approved drug products and includes evaluations of therapeutic equivalents (generic drugs).

D) Incorrect. *The Physician's Desk Reference* is a compilation of annually updated manufacturers' prescribing information (package inserts) on prescription drugs.

51.
A) **Correct.** Trouble opening bottles is a special consideration.

B) Incorrect. Current medications are noted in a patient's profile to check for therapeutic duplications.

C) Incorrect. Current medications are noted in the patient's profile to check for drug duplications.

D) Incorrect. Current medications are noted in a patient's profile to check for adverse reactions.

52.
A) Incorrect. The pharmacist would be responsible.

B) **Correct.** The patient trusted that the pharmacy filled the correct medicine; she would not be responsible for the error.

C) Incorrect. The pharmacy technician is responsible.

D) Incorrect. The place of business is held responsible.

53.
A) Incorrect. The hazard communication plan should include the location of the MSDS.

B) Incorrect. The hazard communication plan should include the location of hazard-related information.

C) Incorrect. The hazard communication plan should include the location of cleaning equipment.

D) **Correct.** The hazard communication plan does not need to discuss worker's compensation claims.

54.
A) Incorrect. A capsule is encapsulated gelatin that is filled with medication.

B) **Correct.** A tablet can be made using a mold.

C) Incorrect. A solution is a liquid.

D) Incorrect. A lotion is a topical solution.

55. A) Incorrect. A water treatment is hydrotherapy.

B) Incorrect. A nerve spasm is a neurospasm.

C) Incorrect. Head pain is encephalodynia.

D) Correct. The suffix –*centesis* provides the clue, meaning surgical puncture for removal of fluid.

56. A) Incorrect. Medicare is a government plan for Americans over sixty-five years old or who meet certain other criteria.

B) Correct. Private employee group health plans are not government plans.

C) Incorrect. Medicaid is a government health plan for Americans whose income is below the poverty level or who meet certain other criteria.

D) Incorrect. TRICARE is a government health plan for those who presently serve or have served in the military.

57.

$$\frac{2}{3} - \frac{1}{5} =$$

$$\frac{2}{3}\left(\frac{5}{5}\right) - \frac{1}{5}\left(\frac{3}{3}\right) =$$

$$\frac{10}{15} - \frac{3}{15}$$

First, multiply each fraction by a factor of 1 to get a common denominator. How do you know which factor of 1 to use? Look at the other fraction and use the number found in that denominator.

$$\frac{10}{15} - \frac{3}{15} = \frac{7}{15}$$

Once the fractions have a common denominator, simply subtract the numerators.

58. A) Incorrect. Sterile compounding is not necessary for compounds taken by mouth.

B) Incorrect. Suppositories are taken rectally; this is not a sterile route.

C) Incorrect. Sublingual administration, in which a medication is dissolved under the tongue, does not require sterile compounding.

D) Correct. Medications administered intravenously are injected into a vein and go directly into the bloodstream, so they require sterile compounding.

59. A) Incorrect. Cocaine is a CII drug.

B) Correct. Marijuana is still considered a CI drug.

C) Incorrect. Oxycodone is a CII drug.

D) Incorrect. Hydrocodone is considered a CII drug.

60. A) Incorrect. Technicians frequently research monographs.

B) Incorrect. Technicians often seek out more information about the brand or generic names of drugs.

C) Incorrect. Technicians commonly research drug interactions.

D) Correct. Pharmacists, not technicians, usually research peer reviews by experts.

61. A) Incorrect. Working only with those medications and devices approved by the law and of good quality is part of the pharmacy technicians' code of ethics.

B) Incorrect. It is the duty of the pharmacy technician to observe the law, behave morally and ethically, and uphold ethical principles.

C) Incorrect. Networking with relevant organizations is part of the code of ethics.

D) Correct. Only the pharmacist counsels patients.

62. **A) Correct.** The prefix *epi–* means upon or above.

B) Incorrect. The suffix –*al* means pertaining to.

C) Incorrect. The word root *derm* means skin.

D) Incorrect.

63. A) Incorrect. The size of the vial is not determined until after the correct number of pills has been counted out to disperse.

B) Incorrect. The technician determines how many pills to count after removing the bottle from the shelf and checking the NDC number.

C) **Correct.** The NDC number must be checked immediately when removing the bottle from the shelf.

D) Incorrect. The technician verifies the patient's name before taking the bottle off the shelf.

64. A) Incorrect. The prefix *osteo–* means bone.

B) **Correct.** The word root *myel* means muscle.

C) Incorrect. The suffix *–itis* means inflammation of.

D) Incorrect.

65. A) Incorrect. Root cause analysis is used by pharmacies for CQI.

B) **Correct.** Suggestion boxes are not used for CQI.

C) Incorrect: FMEA is used for CQI.

D) Incorrect: FOCUS-PDCA is used for CQI.

66. A) Incorrect. Tier 1 is generic drugs.

B) **Correct.** Tier 2 is for preferred drugs.

C) Incorrect. Tier 3 is for non-preferred drugs.

D) Incorrect. Tier 4 is not a category.

67. A) Incorrect. Blind patients are eligible for Medicaid.

B) Incorrect. Disabled patients are eligible for Medicaid.

C) Incorrect. Those patients who live below the poverty level are eligible for Medicaid.

D) **Correct.** Patients who do not work and who live above the poverty level do not qualify for Medicaid.

68. A) Incorrect. The active ingredient of a drug is vital to its efficacy.

B) **Correct.** The color of a drug does not affect its ability to treat its targeted disease or condition.

C) Incorrect. The dosage of a generic drug must be the same as the brand name drug.

D) Incorrect. The strength of a drug is another factor crucial to that drug's efficacy.

69. A) **Correct.** B is used for a hospital or clinic.

B) Incorrect. M is used for a mid-level practitioner.

C) Incorrect. L is used for reverse distributor.

D) Incorrect. A is used for older entities.

70. A) Incorrect. This number is too high.

B) Incorrect. This number is too low.

C) Incorrect. This number is also too low.

D) **Correct.** These quantities are equivalent.

71. A) **Correct.** Although the FDA is involved in non-sterile compounding due to the routes of administration, sterile compounding is considered a part of pharmacy practice and does not fall under the agency's authority.

B) Incorrect. Air quality is an important part of USP 797 because particulates in the air must not contaminate the sterile environment.

C) Incorrect. USP 797 provides very stringent guidelines on the stability and sterilization of CSPs.

D) Incorrect. Because USP 797 is revised often, continuing education is needed to keep personnel up to date on policies and procedures.

72. A) Incorrect. The USP was not made a legal standard in 1901.

B) Incorrect. The USP was not made a legal standard in 1938.

C) **Correct.** The USP was made a legal standard in 1907.

D) Incorrect. The USP was not made a legal standard in 1975.

73. A) Incorrect. This arithmetic is a step in the DEA formula.

B) Incorrect. The first letter of the practitioner's last name should match the second letter in the DEA number.

C) Correct. The first, third, and fifth numbers should be added together, but not multiplied by 2.

D) Incorrect. The first letter of the DEA number must delineate a DEA registrant type that is able to write prescriptions.

74. **A) Correct.** Pharmacy technicians usually use tertiary sources in research.

B) Incorrect. While technicians do use secondary sources, these sources are not consulted as frequently as tertiary sources are.

C) Incorrect. Pharmacy technicians do not generally use primary sources for research.

D) Incorrect. Tertiary, secondary, and primary resources denote sources of information used in research.

75. **A) Correct.** The PCN is used by PBMs for network benefit routing and may change depending on what benefit is being billed.

B) Incorrect. The group number directs the claim to the specific insurance benefits for that group, which is a collection of people with similar benefits packages.

C) Incorrect. The BIN number directs the claim to the correct third-party provider.

D) Incorrect. The cardholder name indicates the beneficiary who receives the health insurance. The patient may not be the beneficiary.

76. A) Incorrect. Drugs in the same drug class must have the same targeted mechanism in order to concentrate the drugs' properties in the body as expected.

B) Incorrect. Having the same mode of action is important for uniformity and dependability of treatment among drugs in the same class.

C) Correct. Drugs do not have to have the same active ingredient to be in the same drug class since each drug is chemically different.

D) Incorrect. Drugs in the same drug class must have similar molecular structures even if their active ingredients vary.

77. A) Incorrect. This quantity is too low.

B) Correct. Since 1 dram can be 4 or 5 mls, 8 tablespoonful can be converted to 24 drams.

C) Incorrect. This quantity is too low.

D) Incorrect. This quantity is too high.

78. A) Incorrect. Refill too soon is a reason for a rejected claim.

B) Incorrect. Claims may be rejected due to quantity limits exceeded.

C) Correct. If there was no refill available on the prescription, the claim would not have been sent in the first place.

D) Incorrect. If prior authorization is required, a claim may be rejected.

79. A) Incorrect. The ASP is based on the selling price data from manufacturers as well as volume discounts and price concessions.

B) Correct. The WAC is the list price that the manufacturer sells the drug to the wholesaler.

C) Incorrect. The AWP is the average price paid to manufacturers from the wholesalers, who only distribute to retail pharmacies.

D) Incorrect. The FUL is the maximum of federal matching funds the federal government will pay to state Medicaid programs for eligible drugs.

80.

$2\frac{1}{3} =$ $\frac{2 \times 3}{3} + \frac{1}{3} =$ $\frac{7}{3}$	This is a fraction subtraction problem with a mixed number, so the first step is to convert the mixed number to an improper fraction.
$\frac{7}{3} \times \frac{2}{2} = \frac{14}{6}$ $\frac{3}{2} \times \frac{3}{3} = \frac{9}{6}$	Next, convert each fraction so they share a common denominator.
$\frac{14}{6} - \frac{9}{6} = \frac{5}{6}$	Now, subtract the fractions by subtracting the numerators.

81. **A)** **Correct.** The suffixes listed distinguish corticosteroids, which reduce inflammation; they do not work with the cardiovascular system.

B) Incorrect. Corticosteroids can work with the respiratory system to reduce lung inflammation.

C) Incorrect. Corticosteroids can work with the immune system too, by reducing inflammation in autoimmune diseases.

D) Incorrect. Corticosteroids can also work with the musculoskeletal system, reducing joint inflammation.

82. A) Incorrect. A virus is an infective agent capable of multiplying in the cells of a living host.

B) Incorrect. Fungi decompose and absorb organic material.

C) **Correct.** A bacterium can become a pyrogen if introduced into the bloodstream.

D) Incorrect. Bacteria can grow by the millions anywhere, including on soft surface areas.

83. A) Incorrect. Point of service is a type of health insurance plan.

B) Incorrect. Dispensing fees are a fee pharmacies charge for professional services.

C) Incorrect. APC is ambulatory payment classification.

D) **Correct.** Retrospective payments are also fee-for-service.

84. A) Incorrect. Use of another person's card is considered fraud.

B) **Correct.** Billing a claim with the correct information on it is not fraud.

C) Billing for services not rendered is fraud.

D) Altering monetary amounts on a claim is fraud.

85. A) Incorrect. Drugs with the suffix –*cillin*, like penicillin, are antibiotics, which kill bacteria.

B) **Correct.** Drugs with the suffix –*vir* are antivirals.

C) Incorrect. Drugs with the suffix –*mycin*, like erythromycin, are also antibiotics, which kill bacteria.

D) Incorrect. Drugs with the suffix –*cycline*, like doxycycline, are antibiotics too, which kill bacteria.

86. A) Incorrect. 2.5 pints does not equal 1500 mL.

B) Incorrect. 2.5 pints does not equal 960 mL.

C) **Correct.** 2.5 pints does equal 1200 mL.

D) Incorrect. 2.5 pints does not equal 960 mL.

87. **A)** **Correct.** A picture of the drug is not required on a prescription label.

B) Incorrect. The order number must be displayed on the prescription label.

C) Incorrect. The prescription label must include the directions for use.

D) Incorrect. The patient's name must be on the prescription label.

88. A) Incorrect. The CII drug order information is recorded on a CII perpetual inventory log.

B) **Correct.** Patient names are not listed on the perpetual inventory log.

C) Incorrect. The CII drug order should be recorded on the log when received from the manufacturer.

D) Incorrect. The balance of the quantity is always logged after each drug transaction carried out for the specific CII drug.

89. **A)** **Correct.** Technicians may not recap, bend, or break contaminated needles or other sharps.

B) Incorrect. This is a safety guideline.

C) Incorrect. This is a safety guideline.

D) Incorrect. This is a safety guideline.

CONTINUE

90. $\dfrac{1}{2} \times \dfrac{8}{8} = \dfrac{8}{16}$

$\dfrac{7}{4} \times \dfrac{4}{4} = \dfrac{28}{16}$

$\dfrac{9}{16} + \dfrac{8}{16} + \dfrac{28}{16} =$

$\dfrac{45}{16}$

For this fraction addition problem, we need to find a common denominator. Notice that 2 and 4 are both factors of 16, so 16 can be the common denominator.

FOUR: Practice Test Four

READ THE QUESTION CAREFULLY AND CHOOSE THE MOST CORRECT ANSWER, OR WORK THE PROBLEM.

1. The systolic reading in blood pressure measures
    A) the heart when it relaxes and fills back up with blood.
    B) the number of heart beats per minute.
    C) the pressure as the heart pumps blood through the body.
    D) the oxygen level in the coronary arteries.

2. Which is NOT a guideline for the emergency dispensing of a CII prescription?
    A) The quantity dispensed can only be enough to sustain the patient during the emergency time period.
    B) A physician cannot ask the pharmacist to dispense a CII prescription in an emergency if the physician is out of town.
    C) The pharmacist must document on the prescription that it was dispensed in an emergency.
    D) The hard copy must be attached and filed with the record of the oral prescription.

3. Sabrina has $\frac{2}{3}$ of a can of red paint. Her friend Amos has $\frac{1}{6}$ of a can. How much red paint do they have combined?

4. Which is NOT a work practice control as defined by OSHA?
    A) universal precautions
    B) biohazard symbols
    C) proper disinfection procedures
    D) proper handling of spills

5. Triglycerides are
    A) what calories are converted to in the body.
    B) the "bad" cholesterol in the body.
    C) the "good" cholesterol in the body.
    D) the waxy substance derived from lipids.

6. Drugs with the suffix –pril are
    A) calcium channel blockers.
    B) beta-blockers.
    C) fibric acid.
    D) ACE inhibitors.

7. Vasodilators

  A) reduce cholesterol in the body.

  B) thin the blood.

  C) treat severe high blood pressure.

  D) are diuretics.

8. If pharmacy technicians have any questions about dispensing a controlled substance medication, they should

  A) ask the lead pharmacy technician.

  B) enter the prescription into the software system and see if the insurance approves or rejects it.

  C) dispense the medication at their own risk.

  D) ask the pharmacist for guidance.

9. What should always be placed on CIII – CV prescriptions when filing hard copies in a two-file system?

  A) a red *X* stamped in the lower left-hand corner

  B) a red *C* stamped in the lower left-hand corner

  C) a red *C* stamped in the lower right-hand corner

  D) a red *X* stamped in the lower right-hand corner

10. Which is NOT a cytotoxic disposal guideline?

  A) Cytotoxic waste must be incinerated at a temperature of 400 to 800 degrees Celsius.

  B) A spill kit must be readily available where hazardous and cytotoxic agents are stored and prepared.

  C) Cytotoxic waste must be separated from biohazardous waste.

  D) Waste such as tubing and PPEs must be placed in leak-proof and tear-resistant containers identified with the cytotoxic symbol.

11. What is the product of $\frac{1}{12}$ and $\frac{6}{8}$?

12. Infection control is a sub-practice of

  A) epidemiology.

  B) biology.

  C) immunology.

  D) ecology.

13. Which is NOT a class of neurons?

  A) central neurons

  B) efferent neurons

  C) interneurons

  D) afferent neurons

14. Which is NOT a trigger for migraines?

  A) food or drink

  B) hormones

  C) stress

  D) obesity

15. In the event of a spill, which of the following is NOT a required step?

  A) rinse area well with clean water

  B) add acidic detergent to water

  C) garb up with PPEs

  D) complete the spill report card

16. Find $\frac{7}{8} \div \frac{1}{4}$.

17. What must the pharmacy technician immediately do if DEA agents identify themselves for an inspection?

  A) retrieve all records needed for the inspection

  B) allow the agents into the pharmacy and start showing them around

  C) show the inspectors where the file system is located

  D refer the agents to the pharmacist-in-charge

18. What is NOT performed in the anteroom?

    A) label preparation

    B) compounding under the laminar airflow workbench

    C) garbing up

    D) order entry

19. Which is NOT a cognition-enhancing medication?

    A) donepezil

    B) memantine

    C) diazepam

    D) galantamine

20. What is the quotient of $\frac{2}{5} \div 1\frac{1}{5}$?

21. According to the DEA, what is the main requirement for a pharmacy or physician's office to e-prescribe controlled substances?

    A) a manual signature from the physician

    B) The patient must have an ER.

    C) Both entities (the pharmacy and doctor's office) must be certified and audited to do so by a third-party auditor.

    D) Both entities (the pharmacy and doctor's office) must be authorized by the state BOP.

22. Which drug class suffix refers to benzodiazepines?

    A) –artan

    B) –pam

    C) –ine

    D) –olol

23. Find the sum of 17.07 and 2.52.

24. Which of the following does NOT fall under the purview of a DUR?

    A) duplicate therapies

    B) substitution of a different generic if the usual generic medication is not available

    C) drug-disease contraindications

    D) drug allergies

25. The bones and joints of the skeletal system are responsible for doing all of the following EXCEPT

    A) allowing movement.

    B) storing fat.

    C) metabolizing sugar.

    D) creating blood cells.

26. Which of the following immunizations is NOT likely to be offered to an institutional pharmacy technician?

    A) flu shot

    B) pneumonia shot

    C) hepatitis B vaccination

    D) HPV vaccination

27. Jeannette has 7.4 gallons of gas in her tank. After driving, she has 6.8 gallons. How many gallons of gas did she use?

28. Which is NOT a purpose of the PDMP?

    A) to track and deter patients from taking narcotics who have chronic pain

    B) to support access to legitimate medical use of controlled substances

    C) to identify and deter or prevent drug abuse and diversion

    D) to inform public health initiatives through outlining use and abuse trends

29. Muscles can contract through motor neurons in all these ways EXCEPT

   A) calcification.

   B) isotonic movements.

   C) isometric movements.

   D) muscle tone.

30. All these drugs are considered NSAIDs EXCEPT

   A) aspirin.

   B) acetaminophen.

   C) naproxen.

   D) ibuprofen.

31. What is the product of 0.25 and 1.4?

32. Which is considered an ergonomic hazard?

   A) incorrect shoes without slip-resistant soles

   B) incorrect lifting technique

   C) incorrect workplace design

   D) incorrect spill clean up

33. What is the definition of pressure differentiation?

   A) control of the environment

   B) any environment that takes in more than 35,200 particulates

   C) change in pressure between the clean room and anteroom

   D) an ISO 5 environment

34. Which of the following is NOT a way to control theft and drug diversion?

   A) keeping CII drugs alongside non-control drugs

   B) controlled accessibility

   C) self-locking doors

   D) electronic alarm systems

35. Which responsibility is NOT considered a daily task?

   A) general clean up

   B) filing hard copies of prescriptions

   C) cycle counts

   D) returning used stock bottles to shelves

36. Find $0.8 \div 0.2$.

37. Which of these is NOT an OSHA requirement for a fire safety plan?

   A) written procedures that diagram exit and escape routes

   B) regular inspection of fire equipment

   C) proper training for all employees in fire prevention strategies and fire drills

   D) safety plans may be distributed to staff

38. Which is NOT required on DEA Form 222 when a pharmacist is ordering CII drugs?

   A) order number

   B) number of packages

   C) size of package

   D) doctor's DEA number

39. All these drugs are opioid analgesics EXCEPT

   A) oxycodone.

   B) tramadol.

   C) fentanyl.

   D) cocaine.

40. Which profession does NOT have prescribing authority?

   A) nurse practitioners

   B) pharmacy technicians

   C) physicians

   D) psychiatrists

41. Major factors of ALARA consist of all of these EXCEPT

  A) time.

  B) distance.

  C) weight.

  D) shielding.

42. A clean room environment must not allow more than how many particles in?

  A) 3,520,000

  B) 35,200

  C) 352

  D) 3,500

43. The GI tract is composed of everything EXCEPT the

  A) stomach.

  B) kidneys.

  C) intestines.

  D) esophagus.

44. What do antiemetics do?

  A) treat vomiting

  B) treat diarrhea

  C) treat constipation

  D) treat gas

45. Which of the following is NOT a requirement of the CMEA?

  A) A 30-day supply of medication containing ephedrine or pseudoephedrine is limited to 9 grams per 30-day supply in retail environments.

  B) Sellers must obtain self-certification.

  C) Patients are required to have a prescription to receive ephedrine and pseudoephedrine.

  D) Selling products containing ephedrine or pseudoephedrine requires employee training.

46. Which is NOT a symptom of Crohn's disease?

  A) malnutrition

  B) weight gain

  C) anemia

  D) fatigue

47. Find the quotient when 40 is divided by 0.25.

48. Inventory management consists of all of the following tasks EXCEPT

  A) distribution.

  B) disposal of products.

  C) proper inventory storage.

  D) ringing up customers.

49. What is NOT a reason that unit-dose medications are used in institutional pharmacy?

  A) to cut costs

  B) for efficiency

  C) so technicians do not need to count out pills

  D) for easier inventory in automated dispensing machines

50. There are 90 voters in a room, and each is either a Democrat or a Republican. The ratio of Democrats to Republicans is 5:4. How many Republicans are there?

51. Scope of practice

  A) is the FDA's safety and adverse event reporting program.

  B) is a guiding sense of obligation.

  C) is a set of moral principles.

  D) is defined by whether the practitioner can diagnose or treat a condition and if so, how that determines the prescriptive authority the practitioner has per state law.

52. Which of these medications is a proton pump inhibitor?

A) misoprostol

B) famotidine

C) sucralfate

D) pantoprazole

53. Which drug is NOT considered a controlled substance?

A) hallucinogens

B) NSAIDs

C) opioids

D) sedatives

54. The ratio of students to teachers in a school is 15:1. If there are 38 teachers, how many students attend the school?

55. PAR levels

A) consist of keeping track of the minimum and maximum level of a particular drug to be available at all times.

B) are not maintained in the pharmacy through the use of inventory systems.

C) classify drugs based on importance.

D) cannot be adjusted periodically depending on the supply and demand of the drug.

56. What is beyond-use dating?

A) the expiration date on the medication vial

B) the expiration date on the IV fluid

C) the expiration date after the CSP has been prepared per manufacturer's instructions

D) the expiration date after the CSP has been prepared if not refrigerated

57. If 35 : 5 :: 49 : x, find x.

58. Whom should the pharmacist contact first if the theft or loss of a controlled substance occurs?

A) the local police

B) the DEA

C) the BOP

D) the company CEO

59. A Class II recall occurs when

A) the product is not likely to cause an adverse event but has violated FDA regulations.

B) a product has a minor violation that does not require legal action, but the product still must be removed from the market to correct the violation.

C) the product may cause temporary health problems, and there is a remote probability of an adverse health event.

D) there is a probability that the use of or exposure to the product could cause an adverse event, health consequences, or death.

60. The pancreas releases which hormone?

A) melatonin

B) thyroxine

C) glucagon

D) epinephrine

61. DEA numbers are comprised of

A) two letters and seven numbers.

B) three letters, six numbers, and one check digit.

C) two letters, six numbers, and one check digit.

D) two letters, five numbers, and two check digits.

62. Which of the following is the most common ratio of pharmacy technicians to each pharmacist?

    A) 6:1

    B) 5:1

    C) 3:1

    D) 2:1

63. Which regulating agency does NOT enforce laws and regulations under the CSA?

    A) DEA

    B) FDA

    C) EPA

    D) the Department of Health and Human Services

64. Which of the following is NOT required to be on a label in hospital pharmacy?

    A) patient's address

    B) patient's name

    C) patient's room number

    D) patient's medical record number

65. Which of the following is NOT a reason for drug shortages?

    A) The vendor does not want to stock the drug anymore.

    B) natural disasters

    C) changes in the formulation of the drug

    D) regulatory issues

66. What is the lowest strength of isopropyl alcohol required for sterilization in the clean room?

    A) 70 percent

    B) 90 percent

    C) 50 percent

    D) 80 percent

67. A train traveling 120 miles takes 3 hours to get to its destination. How long will it take for the train to travel 180 miles?

68. What do mineralocorticoids do?

    A) regulate glucose

    B) influence salt and water balances

    C) release adrenalin

    D) replace hormone

69. A consumer should not purchase drugs from an online seller if

    A) the website requires a prescription from a doctor before dispensing.

    B) the website has accurate contact information available.

    C) authenticity is validated in regard to certification of the website.

    D) the website contains poor grammar and other mistakes.

70. Which fluid is considered an isotonic solution?

    A) 0.45 percent Normal Saline (1/2NS)

    B) Dextrose 5 percent (D5)

    C) Lactated Ringer's (LR)

    D) bacteriostatic water

71. Which controlled substance is considered a CII drug?

    A) tranquilizers

    B) anabolic steroids

    C) opioids

    D) heroin

72. Greta and Max sell cable subscriptions. In a given month, Greta sells 45 subscriptions and Max sells 51. If 240 total subscriptions were sold in that month, what percent were NOT sold by Greta or Max?

73. Which is a system of purchasing in which the pharmacy and a single wholesaler establish a relationship?

A) prime vendor purchasing

B) special ordering

C) wholesaler purchasing

D) direct purchasing

74. Want books are used for all of the following EXCEPT

A) special ordering.

B) uncommon drugs not normally stocked in the pharmacy but needed for a specific patient.

C) in situations when the pharmacy prematurely runs out of the drug due to high demand, and regular order day is still a few days away.

D) when the drug is running low and the regular weekly order will not be delivered until the next morning.

75. Which is NOT a type of manufactured insulin?

A) lispro

B) detemir

C) glargine

D) dulaglutide

76. One acre of wheat requires 500 gallons of water. How many acres can be watered with 2600 gallons?

77. Which pharmacy automation is used to make CSPs without manual touch by a technician?

A) web-based compliance and disease management tracking systems

B) IV and TPN compounding devices

C) barcode administration technology

D) carousel technology

78. Which DEA form is used for DEA registration?

A) DEA Form 222

B) DEA Form 224

C) DEA Form 106

D) DEA Form 41

79. Which risk level covers preparing multiple CSPs for one specific patient?

A) Level 2

B) Level 1

C) Level 3

D) There is no risk associated with this task.

80. 45 is 15% of what number?

81. When returning a drug to the vendor, all of the following information is required on the return form EXCEPT

A) the item order number.

B) the reason for returning the item.

C) the pharmacy technician's certification number.

D) the order purchase number.

82. Which is NOT a hormone replacement drug?

A) levothyroxine

B) propylthiouracil

C) sitagliptin

D) estrogen

83. Which is NOT a factor in chemical degradation?

A) change in pH

B) change in quantity

C) change in temperature

D) change in drug structure

84. The pharmacy technician is responsible for all the responsibilities involving INDs EXCEPT which of the following?

   A)   inventory management

   B)   handling

   C)   preparing

   D)   ordering

85. Jim spent 30% of his paycheck at the fair. He spent $15 for a hat, $30 for a shirt, and $20 playing games. How much was his check? (Round to nearest dollar.)

86. The DEA formula has all of the following characteristics EXCEPT

   A)   the first letter is the DEA registrant number.

   B)   the second letter is the first letter of the last name of the prescriber.

   C)   The first, second, and third numbers are added together and multiplied by 2.

   D)   The second, fourth, and sixth numbers are added together; then the sum is multiplied by 2.

87. Which is NOT required after receiving an order from a vendor?

   A)   checking each individual drug ordered and comparing the invoices and statements received with what was sent from the vendor

   B)   having the pharmacist sign the invoices on non-controlled drugs

   C)   placing the correct vendor stickers that state the item number on the correct stock bottle for future ordering

   D)   signing and dating the invoices and filing them accordingly

88. What percent of 65 is 39?

89. Which of the following is NOT true about stocking drugs?

   A)   Technicians must be knowledgeable about the arrangement of the drug supply.

   B)   Drugs are separated by their routes of administration.

   C)   All pharmacies arrange drugs on the shelf alphabetically by brand name.

   D)   Refrigerated drugs must be stored in the refrigerator as soon as possible.

90. What is the flow rate of an IV infusion?

   A)   medication drops per minute or per hour

   B)   the quantity needed for infusion

   C)   the dosing rate

   D)   the therapeutic dose

PRACTICE TEST FOUR ANSWER KEY

1.

A) Incorrect. Diastolic readings measure when the heart relaxes and fills with blood.

B) Incorrect. The number of beats per minute is the pulse.

C) Correct. Systolic readings measure the pressure as the heart pumps blood through the body.

D) Incorrect. Oxygen levels are not measured by systolic readings. (They can be measured with a blood test or with the use of a device called a pulse oximeter.)

2.

A) Incorrect. One guideline for emergency dispensing is that the quantity dispensed may only sustain the patient during the emergency time period.

B) Correct. A physician can emergency dispense a CII prescription if he or she is out of town.

C) Incorrect. The pharmacist must document on the prescription that it is an emergency situation.

D) Incorrect. The hard copy must be attached to the record of the oral prescription.

3.

$$\frac{2}{3} \times \frac{2}{2} = \frac{4}{6}$$

To add fractions, make sure that they have a common denominator. Since 3 is a factor of 6, 6 can be the common denominator.

$$\frac{4}{6} + \frac{1}{6} =$$
$$\frac{5}{6} \text{ of a can}$$

Now, add the numerators.

4.

A) Incorrect. Work practice controls include universal precautions.

B) Correct. Biohazard symbols are engineering controls.

C) Incorrect. Work practice controls include proper disinfection procedures.

D) Incorrect. Work practice controls include proper handling of spills.

5.

A) Correct. Triglycerides are what calories are converted to in the body.

B) Incorrect. "Bad" cholesterol is LDL.

C) Incorrect. "Good" cholesterol is HDL.

D) Incorrect. The waxy substance derived from lipids is cholesterol.

6.

A) Incorrect. Calcium channel blockers have the –*pine* suffix.

B) Incorrect. Beta-blockers have the –*olol* suffix.

C) Incorrect. Fibric acid derivatives, such as fenofibrate (Tricor) and gemfibrozil (Lopid), reduce cholesterol.

D) Correct. ACE inhibitors, such as benazepril, fosinopril, and quinapril, indeed have the –*pril* suffix.

7.

A) Incorrect. HMG-CoA reductase inhibitors are used to reduce cholesterol in the body by inhibiting its production.

B) Incorrect. Blood thinners, such as warfarin and enoxaparin, thin the blood.

C) Correct. Vasodilators treat severely high blood pressure.

D) Incorrect. Diuretics, such as furosemide and spironolactone, make you urinate more frequently.

8.

A) Incorrect. Pharmacy technicians should direct questions about controlled substances directly to the pharmacist, not the lead technician.

B) Incorrect. Questions about controlled substances should first be referred to the pharmacist, not to the insurance company.

C) Incorrect. Pharmacy technicians should never fill controlled substances at their own risk.

D) Correct. The pharmacist can fill a controlled substance at his or her discretion, so if the technician has any questions about a controlled substance, they should direct it to the pharmacist.

9.

A) Incorrect. A red *X* in the lower left-hand corner is not required.

B) Incorrect. A red *C* in the lower left-hand corner is not correct.

C) **Correct.** A red *C* in the right-hand corner is required.

D) Incorrect. A red *X* in the lower right-hand corner is incorrect.

10.

A) **Correct.** Cytotoxic waste must be incinerated at a temperature of 800 to 1200 degrees Celsius, not 400 to 800 degrees Celsius.

B) Incorrect. It is true that a spill kit must be readily available where hazardous and cytotoxic agents are stored and prepared.

C) Incorrect. One guideline for cytotoxic waste disposal is that it must be separated from biohazardous waste.

D) Incorrect. Waste such as tubing and PPEs must be placed in leak-proof and tear-resistant containers identified with the cytotoxic symbol.

11.

$\frac{1}{12} \times \frac{6}{8} =$ $\frac{6}{96} = \mathbf{\frac{1}{16}}$	Simply multiply the numerators together and the denominators together, then reduce.
$\frac{1}{12} \times \frac{6}{8} =$ $\frac{1}{12} \times \frac{3}{4} =$ $\frac{3}{48} = \mathbf{\frac{1}{16}}$	Sometimes it's easier to reduce fractions before multiplying if you can.

12.

A) **Correct.** Epidemiology is the branch of medicine that addresses disease control.

B) Incorrect. Biology is the study of life.

C) Incorrect. Immunology is the study of the immune system.

D) Incorrect. Ecology is a branch of biology that deals with the relations of organisms to one another.

13.

A) **Correct.** *Central* is not an actual class of neurons, though it can be confused with the central nervous system.

B) Incorrect. Efferent neurons are motor neurons.

C) Incorrect. Interneurons form complex networks in the CNS.

D) Incorrect. Afferent neurons transport signals from receptors to the CNS.

14.

A) Incorrect. Various types of food or drink can indeed trigger a migraine.

B) Incorrect. Hormonal changes can also trigger a migraine.

C) Incorrect. Stress too can trigger a migraine.

D) **Correct.** Obesity is not a known trigger for a migraine.

15.

A) Incorrect. Pharmacy technicians must use clean water to rinse the area thoroughly.

B) **Correct.** Alkali, not acidic, detergent should be added to water.

C) Incorrect. Garbing with PPEs is required.

D) Incorrect. It is essential to complete a spill report.

16.

$\frac{7}{8} \div \frac{1}{4} =$ $\frac{7}{8} \times \frac{4}{1} = \frac{28}{8} = \mathbf{\frac{7}{2}}$	For a fraction division problem, invert the second fraction and then multiply and reduce.

17.

A) Incorrect. Pharmacy technicians do not retrieve records for the inspectors.

B) Incorrect. Pharmacy technicians do not show the inspectors around the pharmacy.

C) Incorrect. Pharmacy technicians do not show the inspectors where the files are located.

D) **Correct.** Pharmacy technicians should immediately refer the inspectors to the pharmacist-in-charge.

18.

A) Incorrect. Labels can be prepared in the anteroom.

B) **Correct.** The laminar airflow workbench is in the clean room.

C) Incorrect. Garbing up is done in the anteroom.

D) Incorrect. Order entry is done in the anteroom unless the facility puts a specialized computer in the clean room.

19. A) Incorrect. Donepezil is a cognition-enhancing medication.

B) Incorrect. Memantine is also a cognition-enhancing medication.

C) Correct. Diazepam is a benzodiazepine.

D) Incorrect. Galantamine is another cognition-enhancing medication.

20.

$$1\frac{1}{5} =$$

$$\frac{5 \times 1}{5} + \frac{1}{5} = \frac{6}{5}$$

$$\frac{2}{5} \div \frac{6}{5} =$$

$$\frac{2}{5} \times \frac{5}{6} = \frac{10}{30} = \frac{1}{3}$$

This is a fraction division problem, so the first step is to convert the mixed number to an improper fraction.

Now, divide the fractions. Remember to invert the second fraction, and then multiply normally.

21. A) Incorrect. The prescription is signed electronically if e-prescribe is allowed.

B) Incorrect. The patient can have an EHR, but the physician still may not have certification to e-prescribe controlled substances.

C) Correct. The entities (pharmacy and doctor's office) must be certified and audited to allow controlled substance e-prescribing by a third-party auditor.

D) Incorrect. Even if permitted by the state BOP, both the pharmacy and doctor's office must have the correct authorization and certification from a third-party auditor in order to e-prescribe.

22. A) Incorrect. –*artan* is the drug class suffix for angiotensin II receptor blockers (A2RBs).

B) Correct. –*pam* is the drug class suffix for benzodiazepines.

C) Incorrect. –*ine* is not a drug class suffix but is used in chemistry to denote specific substances.

D) Incorrect. –*olol* is the drug class suffix for beta-blockers or beta-adrenergic blocking agents.

23.

$$\begin{array}{r} 17.07 \\ + \ \ 2.52 \\ \hline = \mathbf{19.59} \end{array}$$

Line up the decimals and add the numerals together.

24. A) Incorrect. DURs identify drug therapies.

B) Correct. The third-party payer will not know if a different generic manufacturer needs to be used.

C) Incorrect. A DUR must account for drug-disease contraindications.

D) Incorrect. Drug allergies would appear in a DUR.

25. A) Incorrect. Though movement is the main function of the muscular system, the skeletal system also allows movement.

B) Incorrect. The skeletal system does store fat.

C) Correct. The skeletal system does not metabolize sugar though the muscular system produces adenosine tri-phosphate, the body's most important energy molecule, from glucose.

D) Incorrect. The skeletal system does create blood cells through the process called hematopoiesis.

26. A) Incorrect. It is likely that an institutional pharmacy would require technicians to get a flu shot.

B) Incorrect. Many hospitals suggest all pharmacy staff receive pneumonia shots.

C) Incorrect. An institutional pharmacy technician may be asked to receive a hepatitis B vaccination.

D) Correct. An institutional pharmacy technician would not be asked to receive an HPV immunization.

27.

$$\begin{array}{r} 7.4 \\ - \ 6.8 \\ \hline = \mathbf{0.6 \ gal.} \end{array}$$

Line up the decimals and subtract the numerals.

28. **A)** **Correct.** PDMP is not used to track and/or deter patients who have chronic pain from taking narcotics.

B) Incorrect. PDMP supports access to legitimate medical use of controlled substances.

C) Incorrect. PDMP is used to identify and deter or prevent drug abuse and diversion.

D) Incorrect. PDMP does inform public health initiatives through outlining use and abuse trends.

29. **A)** **Correct.** Calcification does not occur in the muscle's motor neurons.

B) Incorrect. Isotonic movements produce movement.

C) Incorrect. Isometric movements maintain posture and stillness.

D) Incorrect. Muscle tone movements occur naturally and are a constant semi-contraction of the muscle.

30. **A)** Incorrect. Aspirin is an NSAID.

B) **Correct.** Acetaminophen is an analgesic.

C) Incorrect. Naproxen is an NSAID.

D) Incorrect. Ibuprofen is an NSAID.

31.

$25 \times 14 = 350$

There are 2 digits after the decimal in 0.25 and one digit after the decimal in 1.4. Therefore the product should have 3 digits after the decimal: **0.350** is the correct answer.

32. **A)** Incorrect. Shoes that have no slip-resistant soles are a physical hazard.

B) Incorrect. Incorrect lifting is physically hazardous.

C) **Correct.** Incorrect workplace design is an ergonomic hazard.

D) Incorrect. Failure to properly clean up a spill would result in a physical hazard.

33. **A)** Incorrect. This term refers to air quality.

B) Incorrect: The anteroom environments permit 35,200 to 3,520,000 airborne particles in.

C) **Correct.** Pressure differentiation refers to the change in pressure between the anteroom and the clean room. This change keeps air particles out of the clean room.

D) Incorrect. This term describes the clean room.

34. **A)** **Correct.** CII drugs must be kept in a safety cabinet under lock and key or password protected.

B) Incorrect. Controlled accessibility is one way to prevent theft and diversion of drugs.

C) Incorrect. Self-locking doors help prevent theft and diversion.

D) Incorrect. Electronic alarm systems help prevent theft and diversion.

35. **A)** Incorrect. General cleaning up should be done daily.

B) Incorrect. Hard copies of prescriptions are filed every day.

C) **Correct.** Cycle counts are done on a monthly basis.

D) Incorrect. Returning stock bottles is a daily task.

36.

$0.8 \div 2$

$8 \div 2 = 4$

Change 0.2 to 2 by moving the decimal one space to the right.

Next, move the decimal one space to the right on the dividend. 0.8 becomes 8.

Now, divide 8 by 2.

37. **A)** Incorrect. OSHA requires that pharmacies develop written procedures that diagram exit and escape routes.

B) Incorrect. OSHA does require that all fire equipment be regularly inspected.

C) Incorrect. OSHA requires that all employees be properly trained in fire prevention strategies and fire drills.

D) **Correct.** Staff may receive copies of safety plans, but OSHA requires that safety plans are visibly posted.

38. **A)** Incorrect. The order number is required.

B)   Incorrect. The number of packages must be specified on the form.

C)   Incorrect. The form must include the size of the package.

D)   Correct. The purchaser's (pharmacist's) DEA number is required, not the doctor's.

39. A)   Incorrect. Oxycodone is an opioid analgesic.

B)   Incorrect. Tramadol is an opioid derivative analgesic.

C)   Incorrect. Fentanyl is an opioid analgesic.

D)   Correct. Cocaine is a local anesthetic.

40. A)   Incorrect. Nurse practitioners do have some prescribing authority.

B)   Correct. Pharmacy technicians do not have prescribing authority.

C)   Incorrect. Physicians have prescribing authority.

D)   Incorrect. Psychiatrists have prescribing authority.

41. A)   Incorrect. Time is a factor in ALARA.

B)   Incorrect. Distance is a factor in ALARA.

C)   Correct. Weight is not a factor in ALARA.

D)   Incorrect. Shielding is a factor in ALARA.

42. A)   Incorrect. This number describes the highest amount of particles allowed in an anteroom environment.

B)   Incorrect. This number also refers to the anteroom environment.

C)   Incorrect. This number is too low. Some particulates will always come through even in the lowest ISO environment.

D)   Correct. The maximum amount of particles allowed in a clean room environment is 3,500.

43. A)   Incorrect. The stomach is part of the digestive system.

B)   Correct. The kidneys are part of the urinary system.

C)   Incorrect. Both the small and large intestines are part of the digestive system.

D)   Incorrect. The esophagus is part of the digestive system.

44. **A)   Correct.** Antiemetics treat vomiting.

B)   Incorrect. Antidiarrheals treat diarrhea.

C)   Incorrect. Laxatives treat constipation.

D)   Incorrect. Antacids treat gas.

45. A)   Incorrect. 30-day supplies are limited to 9 grams in retail environments.

B)   Incorrect. It is true that sellers must obtain self-certification.

C)   Correct. Patients do not need a prescription to purchase products containing ephedrine or pseudoephedrine in most states.

D)   Incorrect. Selling products containing ephedrine or pseudoephedrine requires employee training.

46. A)   Incorrect. Malnutrition is indeed a symptom of Crohn's.

B)   Correct. Weight loss, not gain, is a symptom of Crohn's.

C)   Incorrect. Anemia is also a symptom of Crohn's.

D)   Incorrect. Fatigue is another symptom of Crohn's.

47.

$40 \div 25$	First, change the divisor to a whole number: 0.25 becomes 25.
$4000 \div 25 =$ **160**	Next, change the dividend to match the divisor by moving the decimal two spaces to the right, so 40 becomes 4000. Now divide.

48. A)   Incorrect. Distribution is part of inventory management.

B)   Incorrect. Product disposal is part of inventory management.

C)   Incorrect. Proper inventory storage is part of inventory management.

D) **Correct.** Ringing up customers is not part of inventory management.

49. A) Incorrect. Unit-dosing is used to cut costs.

B) Incorrect. Unit-dosing does improve efficiency.

C) **Correct.** Although it makes work easier for technicians, unit-dosing in hospital pharmacy is not intended to relieve technicians from counting out pills.

D) Incorrect. Unit-dosing facilitates inventory in automated dispensing machines.

50.

$5 + 4 = 9$ Democrats: $\frac{5}{9}$ Republicans: $\frac{4}{9}$	We know that there are 5 Democrats for every 4 Republicans in the room, which means for every 9 people, 4 are Republicans.
$\frac{4}{9} \times 90 =$ **40 Republicans**	If $\frac{4}{9}$ of the 90 voters are republicans, then multiply the fraction by the whole number.

51. A) Incorrect. The FDA's safety and adverse event reporting program is called Medwatch.

B) Incorrect. Principles are a guiding set of obligations.

C) Incorrect. Ethics are a set of moral principles.

D) **Correct.** Scope of practice is defined by whether the practitioner can diagnose or treat a condition and if so, how that determines the prescriptive authority the practitioner has per state law.

52. A) Incorrect. Misoprostol prevents stomach ulcers.

B) Incorrect. Famotidine is a histamine-2 blocker.

C) Incorrect. Sucralfate treats ulcers.

D) **Correct.** Pantoprazole is a proton pump inhibitor.

53. A) Incorrect. Hallucinogens are controlled substances.

B) **Correct.** NSAIDs are not controlled substances.

C) Incorrect. Opioids are controlled substances.

D) Incorrect. Most sedatives are considered controlled substances.

54.

$\frac{15 \text{ students}}{1 \text{ teacher}} \times$ 38 teachers **= 570 students**	To solve this ratio problem, we can simply multiply both sides of the ratio by the desired value to find the number of students that correspond to having 38 teachers.

55. **A)** **Correct.** PAR levels consist of keeping track of the minimum and maximum level of a particular drug to be available at all times.

B) Incorrect. PAR levels can be maintained in the pharmacy through the use of inventory systems.

C) Incorrect. PAR levels do not classify drugs based on importance.

D) Incorrect. PAR levels can be adjusted periodically depending on the supply and demand of the drug.

56. A) Incorrect. After the vial is punctured and reconstituted it starts to degrade; the expiration date changes as a result.

B) Incorrect. IV fluid also starts to degrade after it has been punctured; again, the expiration date changes.

C) **Correct.** The beyond-use date indicates when the medication expires once the medication is compounded per the manufacturer's instructions.

D) Incorrect. Whether a CSP is refrigerated depends on the medication. The wrong temperature may cause a medication to become unstable, so it is crucial to read the instructions for the CSP in question.

57.

$\frac{35}{5} = \frac{49}{x}$	This problem presents two equivalent ratios that can be set up in a fraction equation.
$35x = 49 \times 5$ $x = \mathbf{7}$	You can then cross-multiply to solve for x.

58.

A) Incorrect. The local police should be contacted, but they are not the first contact.

B) Correct. The pharmacist should immediately contact the DEA before anyone else.

C) Incorrect. The BOP should be contacted but not before the DEA.

D) Incorrect. The company CEO should not be contacted.

59.

A) Incorrect. This describes a Class III recall.

B) Incorrect. This describes an FDA market withdrawal.

C) Correct. A Class II recall is when the product may cause temporary health problems, and there is a remote probability of an adverse health event.

D) Incorrect. This describes a Class I recall.

60.

A) Incorrect. Melatonin is released through the pineal body.

B) Incorrect. Thyroxine is released from the thyroid gland.

C) Correct. The alpha-cells in the pancreas release glucagon.

D) Incorrect. Epinephrine is released through the adrenal glands.

61.

A) Incorrect. DEA numbers use two letters, six numbers, and one check digit.

B) Incorrect. DEA numbers only have two letters.

C) Correct. DEA numbers are comprised of two letters, six numbers, and a check digit.

D) Incorrect. DEA numbers only have one check digit, and they have six numbers.

62.

A) Incorrect. The ratio is not 6:1.

B) Incorrect. The ratio is not 5:1.

C) Correct. The ratio is 3:1.

D) Incorrect. The ratio is not 2:1.

63.

A) Incorrect. The DEA does enforce the CSA.

B) Incorrect. The FDA does enforce the CSA.

C) Correct. The EPA does not enforce the CSA.

D) Incorrect. The Department of Health and Human Services does enforce the CSA.

64.

A) Correct. The patient's address is not needed on a hospital label.

B) Incorrect. The patient's name is required on a hospital label.

C) Incorrect. The patient's room number must be listed on a hospital label.

D) Incorrect. The hospital label must display the patient's medical record number.

65.

A) Correct. Drug shortages do not occur because the vendor voluntarily refuses to stock a drug.

B) Incorrect. Natural disasters can cause drug shortages.

C) Incorrect. Formulation changes can cause drug shortages.

D) Incorrect. Regulatory issues can cause drug shortages.

66.

A) Correct. The lowest strength of isopropyl alcohol permitted for sterilization in the clean room is 70 percent.

B) Incorrect. Although 90 percent is available and can be used, the lowest strength permissible is 70 percent.

C) Incorrect. Isopropyl alcohol 50 percent would not effectively disinfect in the clean room; this percentage is too low.

D) Incorrect. There is no such strength as 80 percent isopropyl alcohol.

67.

$$\frac{120 \text{ miles}}{3 \text{ hours}} = \frac{180 \text{ miles}}{x \text{ hours}}$$

Start by setting up the proportion (note that it doesn't matter which value is placed in the numerator or denominator, as long as it is the same on both sides).

120 miles × x hours = 3 hours × 180 miles	Now, solve for the missing quantity through cross–multiplication.
$x = \dfrac{(3\ hours) \times (180\ hours)}{120\ miles}$ **= 4.5 hours**	Now solve the equation.

68.   A)   Incorrect. Glucocorictoids regulate glucose.

      B)   **Correct.** Mineralocorictoids influence salt and water balances.

      C)   Incorrect. The adrenal glands release adrenalin.

      D)   Incorrect. Hormone replacement therapy replaces hormones.

69.   A)   Incorrect. An online seller that requires a prescription from a doctor before dispensing drugs is more reputable.

      B)   Incorrect. An online retailer is more trustworthy if its website has accurate contact information available.

      C)   Incorrect. It may be safer for a consumer to purchase drugs from an online seller if authenticity is validated in regard to certification of the website.

      D)   **Correct.** A consumer should not purchase drugs from an online seller if the website contains poor grammar and other mistakes.

70.   A)   Incorrect. 1/2NS is considered hypertonic.

      B)   Incorrect. Dextrose 5 percent is used for caloric replenishment and is hypotonic.

      C)   **Correct.** Lactated Ringer's is an isotonic solution.

      D)   Incorrect. Bacteriostatic water is not used for IVs.

71.   A)   Incorrect. Tranquilizers are CIV drugs.

      B)   Incorrect. Anabolic steroids are CIII drugs.

      C)   **Correct.** Opioids are CII drugs.

      D)   Incorrect. Heroin is a CI drug.

72.

$percent = \dfrac{part}{whole} = \dfrac{(51 + 45)}{240} =$ $\dfrac{96}{240} = 0.4$ or 40%	You can use the information in the question to figure out what percent-age of subscriptions were sold by Max and Greta.
100% − 40% = **60%**	However, the question asks how many subscriptions *weren't* sold by Max or Greta. If they sold 40%, then the other salespeo-ple sold the rest.

73.   **A)**   **Correct.** Prime vendor purchasing is a system of purchasing in which a relationship is established between the pharmacy and a single wholesaler.

      B)   Incorrect. Pharmacies use special ordering to obtain specific drugs such as investigational drugs, controlled substances, cytotoxic drugs, and hazardous substances.

      C)   Incorrect. In wholesaler purchasing, many products are purchased from one vendor source.

      D)   Incorrect. Direct purchasing eliminates the need for intermediary and handling fees for drug procurement.

74.   A)   Incorrect. Want books are used for special order items.

      B)   Incorrect. Want books are used for such drugs.

      C)   Incorrect. Want books are used in these situations.

      D)   **Correct.** Want books are not used in these situations.

75.   A)   Incorrect. The brand name for lispro is Humalog/NovoLog.

      B)   Incorrect. The brand name for detemir is Levemir.

      C)   Incorrect. The brand name for glargine is Lantus.

      D)   **Correct.** Dulaglutide's brand name is Trulicity, an antidiabetic, not an insulin.

76.

$\dfrac{1 \text{ acre}}{500 \text{ gal.}} = \dfrac{x \text{ acres}}{2600 \text{ gal.}}$	Set up the equation.
$x \text{ acres} = \dfrac{1 \text{ acre} \times 2600 \text{ gal.}}{500 \text{ gal.}}$ $x = \dfrac{26}{5}$ or **5.2 acres**	Then solve for x.

77. A) Incorrect. Web-based compliance and disease management tracking systems are used for tracking patient compliance and disease management.

B) **Correct.** IV and TPN compounding devices prevent technicians from manually preparing sterile preparations.

C) Incorrect. Barcode administration technology helps prevent medication errors as the nurse must check the barcode on the patient with the barcode on the medication label.

D) Incorrect. Carousel technology reduces a technician's travel time, bending, and reaching in the fill process. The rotating shelving also allows pharmacies to take advantage of space in the pharmacy that is not being utilized.

78. A) Incorrect. DEA Form 222 is used for ordering CII drugs.

B) **Correct.** DEA Form 224 is for DEA registration.

C) Incorrect. DEA Form 106 is used for theft or loss of schedule drugs.

D) Incorrect. DEA Form 41 is for destroying controlled substances.

79. A) **Correct.** Level 2 covers bulk compounding, which consists of preparing multiple CSPs for one patient.

B) Incorrect. Level 1 covers minimal preparations.

C) Incorrect. Level 3 does cover all levels, but focuses on CSPs that are susceptible to contamination.

D) Incorrect. Preparing multiple CSPs for one specific patient falls under risk level 2.

80.

$whole = \dfrac{part}{percent} =$ $\dfrac{45}{0.15} = \mathbf{300}$	Set up the appropriate equation and solve. Don't forget to change 15% to a decimal value.

81. A) Incorrect. The item order number is required on the return form.

B) Incorrect. The return form must include the reason for returning the item.

C) **Correct.** The pharmacy technician's certification number is not required on the return form.

D) Incorrect. The return form must contain the order purchase number.

82. A) Incorrect. Levothyroxine (Synthroid) is indeed a hormone replacement drug.

B) Incorrect. Propylthiouracil (PTU) is also hormone replacement drug.

C) **Correct.** Sitagliptin (Januvia) is used to treat type 2 diabetes.

D) Incorrect. Estrogen is another hormone replacement drug. Some of its brand names are Premarin, Prempro, Climara, and Depo-Estradiol.

83. A) Incorrect. One factor in degradation may be change in pH.

B) **Correct.** A change in quantity will not affect degradation of a CSP.

C) Incorrect. Change in temperature can cause cloudiness, crystallization, and change in potency.

D) Incorrect. Degradation can cause drug structure to become unstable.

84. A) Incorrect. Technicians are responsible for inventory management.

B) Incorrect. Technicians must handle INDs.

C) Incorrect. Preparing INDs is the responsibility of the technician.

D) **Correct.** Technicians are not responsible for ordering INDs; physicians are.

85.

$$whole = \frac{part}{percent} =$$

$$\frac{15 + 30 + 20}{.30} = \mathbf{\$217.00}$$

Set up the appropriate equation and solve.

86.

A) Incorrect. The first letter is the DEA registrant type in the DEA formula.

B) Incorrect. The second letter is the first letter of the last name of the prescriber.

C) Correct. The first, third, and fifth numbers are added together, not the first, second, and third numbers.

D) Incorrect. The second, fourth, and sixth numbers are added together and the sum is then multiplied by 2.

87.

A) Incorrect. Pharmacy technicians must check each individual drug ordered and compare the invoices and statements received with what was sent from the vendor.

B) **Correct.** Pharmacists do not need to sign invoices for non-controlled drugs.

C) Incorrect. Pharmacy technicians must place the correct vendor stickers stating the item number on the correct stock bottle for future ordering.

D) Incorrect. Pharmacy technicians must sign and date the invoices and file them accordingly.

88.

$$percent = \frac{part}{whole} =$$

$$\frac{39}{65} = 0.6 \text{ or } \mathbf{60\%}$$

Set up the appropriate equation and solve.

89.

A) Incorrect. It is true that technicians must be knowledgeable about the arrangement of the drug supply.

B) Incorrect. Drugs are indeed separated by their routes of administration.

C) **Correct.** Not all pharmacies arrange drugs alphabetically by brand name. Some pharmacies arrange drugs by generic name.

D) Incorrect. Refrigerated drugs must be properly stored as soon as possible.

90.

A) **Correct.** The flow rate is the drops per minute or per hour during which a medication is infused.

B) Incorrect. The quantity of a medication needed for infusion is its total volume.

C) Incorrect. The dosing rate is the infusion rate, not the flow rate.

D) Incorrect. The therapeutic dose is the dose of medication that would be effective to treat the disease state.

CPSIA information can be obtained
at www.ICGtesting.com
Printed in the USA
BVHW010214160420
577722BV00012B/329